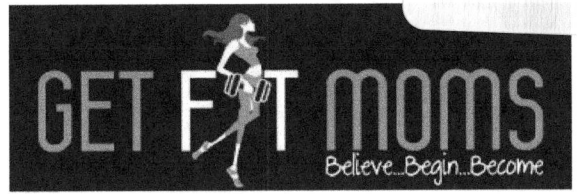

Clean Eats & Treats

Healthy Recipes for the Entire Family

By Kim Lipe & Shauna Cotton

NASM & ISSA Certified Personal Trainer & Certified in Fitness Nutrition

Medical Disclaimer

The information in this work is in no way intended as medical advice or a substitute for medical counseling. This publication contains the opinions and ideas of its author. It is intended to provide helpful and informative material on the subjects addressed in the publication. It is sold with the understanding that the author and publisher are not engaged in rendering medical, health, psychological, or any other kind of personal professional services in the book. If the reader requires personal medical, health, or other assistance or advice, a competent professional should be consulted. The author and publisher specifically disclaim all responsibility for any liability or loss, personal, or otherwise, that is incurred as a consequence, directly or indirectly of the use and application of the contents of this book.

Table of Contents:

Our Story

We know how hectic life can be with a career and raising kids. As a mom, it's hard to find time for yourself. Once you have kids, there is an immediate assumption that you no longer have to take care of yourself. Your job is now to take care of the kids...right?! With the busy life of raising kids, eating healthy and working out go by the way side. The next thing you know, you find yourself stuck in a body that you no longer recognize. And, asking yourself "where did that extra weight come from?"

My mom and I felt this same way! Both of us were in different stages in our lives, mine as a new mom with two little girls and hers now in her mid-40's, but we both felt the same way about ours bodies. Neither of us felt comfortable with our waistlines a little wider and our bottoms a little flatter! After having a few kids and hitting pre-menopause, most of us think, it's pointless now to start eating healthy and working out in hopes to get your 20 year-old body back. My mom and I both had the desire to get back in shape and prove ourselves wrong. We believed we could do this!

My mom, Kim, started working out with a personal trainer at the age of 45. At the time, she learned that she really knew very little about nutrition. My mom raised our family assuming that a home-cooked meal like roast, mashed potatoes, a canned vegetable, bread & butter was the healthiest option. We were a "meat and potatoes" kind of family. My mom didn't stress the importance of eating our fruits and veggies. So, we didn't eat them. And, needless to say I become a very picky eater.

As my mom began working with her trainer, she soon realized that cleaning up her diet was what she needed to do in order to see her progress in the gym. My mom learned how to read food labels and started buying foods that she never would have thought to buy before like *fresh* veggies, fruits, chicken, ground turkey, sweet potatoes. My mom began taking some of our family's favorite recipes and turning them into healthier options.

Eating healthy everyday and working out is now apart of my mom's lifestyle. She lost over 30lbs and went from 30% body fat to 12% body fat within a few years time. Now 53, my mom is a personal trainer, and competes in figure competitions against girls half her age. She is proof that it is never too late to start!

With her amazing results, I was inspired to get in the gym after having my second child. I thought if my mom could have six- pack abs after having 3 kids and now being a grandma of 2, then I could do it too! Living 4 hours apart, we couldn't physically workout together, but she coached me along the way about exercising and nutrition. I began eating fresh fruits and veggies for the first time in my life! I made small changes in my food pantry and learned how to cook healthy for my family without them evening knowing! Reading labels has been one of the most valuable lessons that I have learned from my mom. With her guidance, I lost that last lingering 10lbs that I still had from my first child. I am now in the best shape of my life.

Like my mom, I also become a certified personal trainer and competed in my first fitness competition with my mom! Together, my mom and I created "Get Fit Moms" to inspire other moms that you can live a healthy lifestyle no matter what stage in your life you are! It is still possible to achieve your fitness goals!

It's so important to become a healthy role model for your kids. It starts in the kitchen, by educating and preparing healthy meals for your family. With 140 recipes, we hope this cookbook gives your family a jumpstart to your new healthy lifestyle!

Believe...Begin...Become...a Get Fit Mom (and Family)!

We Believe in You!

Kim & Shauna

Mother-Daughter Personal Training Team

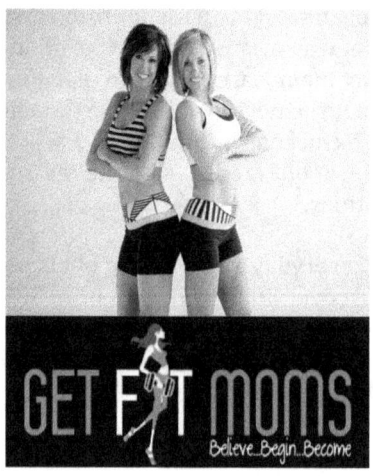

Recipe Index

Success Stories

Ashley lost 30lbs, 9 1/2" total inches and 4% body fat!

My name is Ashley, mother of two, lost 30 lbs. 9 ½ total inches and 4% body fat.

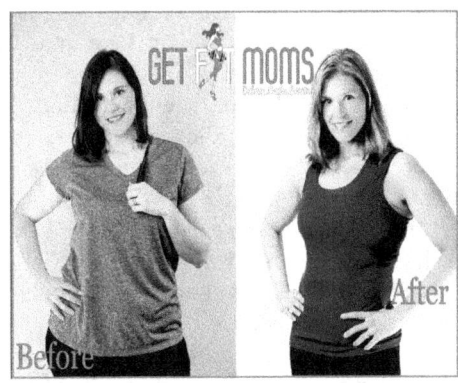

I have struggled with weight my entire life. I was a heavy child, thinned out in high school, gained the first year of college, lost, gained, and so on. I have tried every diet and workout plan imaginable. I would lose for a while and then something wouldn't work and I would get frustrated and give up. Next thing I knew, I was 10 pounds heavier than when I started whatever crazy program I was on.

I was getting close to being the heaviest I had ever been. I heard about Kim through friends and immediately gave her a call. On the very first night, she sat down with me and explained all the ins and outs of the nutrition part of the program. Kim told me how many calories I needed in a day, along with proteins, carbs, and fats. She showed me how to read labels to understand exactly what I was putting in my body. As for the exercise part of the program, Kim has me doing more than I ever imagined I could. I like to say she is the perfect mix of Biggest Losers' Bob and Jillian…she is sweet and supportive like Bob, but can definitely push you like Jillian.

I have never stuck to a program this before. Kim made me understand that this is a life style change and not just something I need to do to be thin, but I need to do this for my health in general. I love the results I am getting with her help. I feel better about myself and have more energy for my everyday life. I have to thank Kim for being there to support and guide me through this journey of a healthier me. I want to thank the girls I work out with at Kim's for providing a fun, motivating place to exercise. I also need to thank my husband, my family and friends for their support and encouragement during this process. All of the help I have received has made this transformation possible!

-Ashley Knisley

Judy, 67 years old, loses 38lbs, 17 ½ total inches and 10% body fat!

My name is Judy Thacker and I'm 67 years old. I have had trouble with my weight all of my life, going up and down. I got up to 167 pounds and I knew I had to do something, but I could not do it on my own. I needed someone who could show me how to eat and exercise correctly to achieve my goals. I have been blessed with good health, but I was not taking very good care of my body. I remember when I was at our local gym, I saw Kim working out. I thought about how much I wished I could get her to train me. Then, one day I saw Kim's Gym and Personal Training Studio in the paper. I quickly called Kim. I am so glad I made that call as I have now lost 38 pounds and 10 percent body fat! As a 66 year old, I am proof it is never to late to start. I want to thank Kim for sharing her vision in helping people get healthy. She is more than a personal trainer, she really cares and wants to help those around her in any way she can. Thank you Kim!

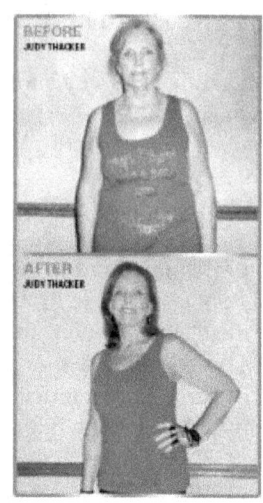

-Judy Thacker

Alisha loses 30lbs and 13 total inches for her wedding!

I feel better about myself and more self-confident. I love how good I feel from eating healthy food! I could not have done any of this without the support of my mom, sister and Kim. I am a picky eater, so finding foods that I enjoy that are healthy was a bit of a challenge. But, I have learned how to overcome my challenges of eating out every weekend and my lack of veggies in my diet. I am so glad that my mom, sister and Kim encouraged me to stick with my healthy lifestyle because I have never felt better about myself.

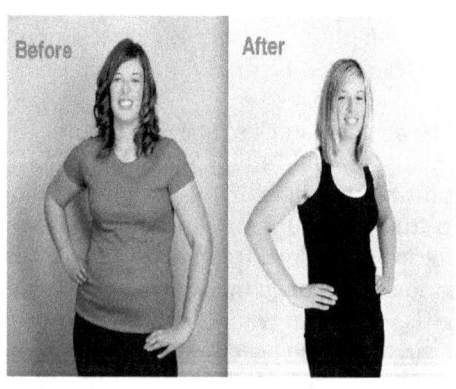

-Alisha Tischhauser

Paula loses 11 lbs and 6% body fat in 28-Day Challenge!

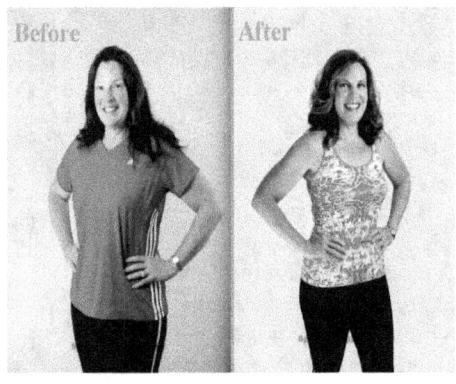

I'm Paula Gephart and I'm 45 years old. I have always struggled with my weight. I was an overweight child, teen and adult. I have tried every fad diet there is and even made up some of my own, only to lose some weight and then gain it all back and then some. I started training with Kim in November 2012. My weight had hit an all time high and I was shocked to find out that I was at 25% body fat. I completed the Get Fit Mom's 28-day challenge and I set a goal for myself to lose 10 lbs. I lost 11 and I am now at 19 % body fat! I love to work out now and I especially love the feeling when I'm finished! I feel proud of myself and I feel proud of all the new friends I have met and worked out with! I love hearing everyone's success story. I can't wait to reach my next goal...my first pull up or another 10 lbs. Whatever it is, I know now with clean healthy eating and the new lifestyle, nothing should be out of reach.   Believe, Begin, Become!

-Paula Gephart

Jordyn, a Freshman in High School, loses 40 lbs and 20½ total inches in 9 months!

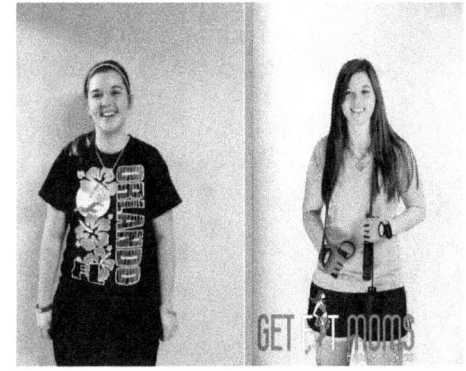

Jordyn began her fitness journey during her 8th grade year. Jordyn and her mom, Crystal, began working out together with Kim. Jordyn had a goal to be fit and healthy by her 8th grade dance. Jordyn did just that! She focused on her nutrition by packing her lunch for school everyday with healthy options. In addition to working out with Kim, she would also take advantage of her P.E. classes to get in a good workout. Jordyn is such a great inspiration to young ladies that you can make a lifestyle change at any age!

-Jordyn Finley

Mandy loses 20lbs, 8 total inches plus 8% body fat!

My name is Mandy Pearson and I am 42 years old. I have always exercised, but never truly got where I wanted to be. I have tried every fad diet, tried every type of workout known to man. In the past I have over-trained and skipped meals. I just couldn't understand why I didn't get where I wanted to be. I couldn't possibly eat any less or exercise any more. I was about to give up.

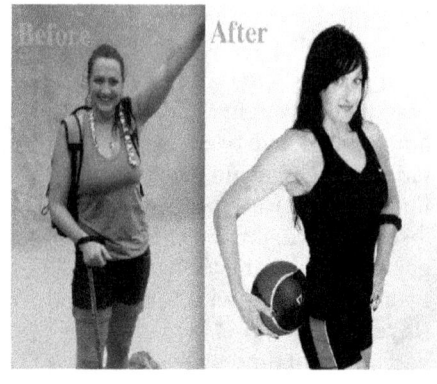

Then, I found Kim Lipe from Get Fit Moms. During our consult, Kim explained to me that it is not a diet. Kim gave me a plan, a new way of eating that I never dreamed would work so perfectly into my lifestyle. I started to eat clean and great things happened. I could not believe how quickly the fat just burned away and how clean I felt inside and out. The confidence I feel just knowing I am controlling what I eat, how I look and feel, is amazing to me. I would have never attempted a plan like this on my own, but Kim gave me easy-to-follow guidelines and sample meals. She also included many recipes that were all "Kim approved" or were her own recipes. She took the guesswork out of the mix. That was my saving grace the first month or so. I followed the plan to a science because I wouldn't have known what to do if I put it in my own hands. Eventually, after several months on this plan, I learned what I can and cannot eat. I simply cannot believe my results. I feel better than I ever have, and that is the absolute truth! They say that abs are made in the kitchen, not the gym, and that results are 70 percent diet and 30 percent exercise. Why didn't anyone tell me that before! My only regret about clean eating is not starting years ago.

Along with the nutritional plan, I started attending Kim's strength training classes. I have always been a cardio, not weight, kind of girl. With my new way of eating and strength training, I have lost flab and replaced it with muscle!

I would highly recommend Kim's recipes. Follow her advice, her recommendations. Follow her workout routines. I guarantee you will be impressed. I thought I had seen and done it all when it came to fitness, but I was wrong.

- Mandy Pearson

The Importance of Nutrition

The body is an extraordinary machine that needs premium fuel to function effectively and efficiently. When your body is functioning at its best, it will automatically burn more calories from its fat stores. By combining a healthy diet with a strength-training program, you will have the body that you have always wanted!

Protein, Carbs & Fats

Protein, carbohydrates and fat are referred to as the macronutrients. To ensure you are burning off body fat and not muscle, you must have all three in your diet to keep your metabolism running effectively. So, why are these nutrients important and how do they affect the body?

Protein = Build Lean Muscle
Protein will help build lean muscle and increase your metabolic rate so you will burn more calories. Protein also helps control hunger and muscle recovery after a workout.

Carbs = Energy
Carbs create energy for the body; therefore, are crucial to have in your diet. Protein & fat are essential to reducing body fat, however, there are no essential carbs. That is because your body can convert protein and fact into carbs. If your goal is to lose weight, complex Carbs are good to eat during the day while Fibrous Carbs are better for your "evening" carbs. This will help you have energy and give you time to burn off all the calories before bedtime.

"Good" Fats = Burn Fat (Monounsaturated & Polyunsaturated also known as EFA's)
Our body needs the "good" fat to maximize your metabolism. Fat acts as a secondary source of energy during training. This energy becomes available soon after carbohydrates stored in the muscles are depleted.

Meal Planning

As a general guide when planning your meals, make sure to consume a protein, carb and fat at each meal. Use the food source charts on pages 23-26 to guide you in your planning.

General Guideline to plan your meals:

Meals/Snacks	Protein	Complex Carbs*	Fibrous Carbs*	Healthy Fats
Meal 1 - breakfast	X	X	X	X
Meal 2 - snack	X	X	X	X
Meal 3 - lunch	X	X	X	X
Meal 4 - snack	X		X	X
Meal 5 - dinner	X		X	X
Meal 6 - snack/optional	X		X	X

*Please note that for Meals 1-3, you can have both kinds of carbs if it fits into your daily carb allowance.

Sugar and Sodium

The reason that we have a difficult time losing weight and keeping it off is not only due to the lack of the macronutrients, but the amount of sugar and sodium we consume. To reduce and eliminate fat, you must limit your sugar & sodium intake. This can be hard because sugar and sodium are found in so many foods! But, if you stay away from processed foods, and focus on eating fresh foods like the ones that we suggest in the upcoming charts, you should find this to not be as much of a problem.

General Guideline for Sugar and Sodium Intake:
Sugar – less than 40 grams per day.
Sodium – less than 2400mg per day.

Guide to Calculating Your Daily Calories

Here is a **_general guideline_** to calculate your daily calories. Many people do not eat enough calories per day when their goal is to lose weight, but they actually need to eat more to lose more of the right foods to achieve their goals. Take your current body weight and times by 10 to give you your daily calorie needs. Again, this is a general starting point for women wanting to lose weight or tone up. If you are extremely active, you may need to increase your calories by multiplying by 12 or 14.

_____ x 10 = _____
Current Body Weight   Daily Caloric Intake

Guide to Calculating Your Daily Protein, Carbs & Fats

After determining your total daily calories, then we break it down into how many of protein, carbs and fats that we need to consume depending on your body type.

3 Body Types:

1. Ectomorph: Long and thin muscles and limbs with lower fat storage, generally slim.
2. Mesomorph: Larger bones, solid torso, wide shoulders, trim waist controlled body fat.
3. Endomorph: Increased fat storage, wider waist, and larger bone structure.

Body Type	Approximate Starting % Protein	Approximate Starting % of Carbs	Approximate Starting % of Fat
Ectomorph	25%	55%	20%
Mesomorph	30%	40%	30%
Endomorph	35%	25%	40%

My Daily Calorie Intake by Nutrient:
Note: we break it down to the grams because that is how food labels read.

PROTEIN _____ x _____ = _____ / 4 = _____
            (Daily Calorie) (% from chart) (Calories needed)   (Grams needed)

CARBS   _____ x _____ = _____ / 4 = _____
            (Daily Calorie) (% from chart) (Calories needed)   (Grams needed)

FATS   _____ x _____ = _____ / 9 = _____
            (Daily Calorie) (% from chart) (Calories needed)   (Grams needed)

21

Food Journaling

The best way to stay focused on your goal, is to write down everything that you eat on a daily basis. Journaling your food will open your eyes as to what foods are truly healthy food choices. Plus, if you have to write it down, you will be less likely to pick up an unhealthy choice. Use this food log to track your foods daily.

	Calories	Protein	Carbs	Fat	Sugar	Sodium
Meal 1						
Meal 2						
Meal 3						
Meal 4						
Meal 5						
Meal 6						
Total						
Goal						
Difference						

Protein	Serving Size	Calories	Protein	Carbs	Fat
Beef Roast/ Tenderloins/ Filets	4 oz	155	23	0	7
Chicken Breast	4 oz	120	25	0	2
Cod	4 oz	120	25	0	1
Low Fat Cottage Cheese	½ cup	90	13	7	1
Egg whites	1 egg	17	4	0	0
Extra Lean Ground Beef	4 oz	150	24	0	5
Extra Lean Ground Turkey Breast	4 oz	130	27	0	2
Flank Steak	4 oz	180	23	0	9
Plain Greek Yogurt	½ cup	67	12	5	0
Extra Lean Ground Chicken	4 oz	120	23	1	2
Lean Bison	4 oz	123	24	0	2
Pork Loin	4 oz	140	26	0	4
Salmon	4 oz	155	22	0	7
Shrimp	4 oz	107	24	0	1
Tilapia	4 oz	110	21	0	3
Top Sirloin Steak	4 oz	150	23	0	5
Tuna	4 oz	140	28	0	2
Turkey Bacon	1 slice	20	3	0	1
Turkey Breast or Cutlets	4 oz	120	26	0	2
Whey Protein Powder	1 scoop	120	20	4	4
Whole Egg	1 egg	74	6	0	5

Complex Carbs	Serving Size	Calories	Protein	Carbs	Fat
Black, Kidney or Pintos Beans	½ cup	100	6	17	1
Brown Rice	½ cup	75	2	17	0
Ezekiel Bread	1 slice	80	4	15	1
Oat Bran	½ up	116	8	31	3
Oatmeal	½ cup	150	5	27	3
P28 Bread	1 slice	130	14	12	4
Red Potato	1	30	3	15	1
Quinoa	¼ cup	170	5	30	3
Sweet Potato	1	86	2	20	0
Wheat Bran	¼ cup	30	2	10	1
Whole Wheat Pasta	2 oz	180	7	41	2
Whole Wheat Bread, Bagel, Pitas and Wraps	1	60	6	8	2
Whole Wheat Cous Cous	¼ cup	150	6	30	1
Rice Cakes	1	35	1	8	0

Fibrous Carbs - Vegetables	Serving Size	Calories	Protein	Carbs	Fat
Asparagus	1 cup	27	3	5	0
Bell Peppers	1 cup	29	1	6	0
Broccoli	1 cup	30	2	6	0
Brussels Sprouts	1 cup	38	3	8	0
Cabbage	1 cup	21	1	5	0
Carrots	1 cup	30	2	8	0
Cauliflower	1 cup	25	2	5	0
Celery	1 cup	14	1	3	0
Cucumber	1 cup	16	0	4	0
Eggplant	1 cup	20	1	5	0
Green Beans	1 cup	44	2	10	0
Kale	1 cup	34	2	7	0
Lettuce	1 cup	5	0	1	0
Mushroom	1 cup	19	1	1	0
Onions	1 cup	67	1	16	0
Peas	1 cup	105	7	18	0
Radish	1 cup	19	1	4	0
Spinach	1 cup	7	1	1	0
Tomato	1 medium	35	1	7	0
Zucchini	1 cup	20	2	4	0

Simple Carbs Fruits	Serving Size	Calories	Protein	Carbs	Fat
Apple	1 medium	100	0	25	0
Banana	1 medium	90	1	23	0
Blueberries	1 cup	83	1	21	0
Dates	1 medium	12	0	3	0
Grapefruit	1 medium	88	2	22	0
Kiwi	1 medium	46	1	11	0
Oranges	1 medium	65	1	15	0
Peaches	1 medium	58	1	14	0
Raspberries	1 cup	64	1	15	0
Strawberries	1 cup	49	1	12	0
Unsweetened Apple Sauce	½ cup	55	0	14	0

Healthy Fats	Serving Size	Calories	Protein	Carbs	Fat
Almond Butter	1 tbsp	95	4	3	8
Avocado	1 medium	250	3	15	23
Better Than Peanut Butter	1 tbsp	50	2	6	1
Coconut Oil	1 tbsp	120	0	0	14
Flaxseed Meal and Oil	1 tbsp	120	0	0	14
Natural Peanut butter	1 tbsp	95	5	4	8
Unsalted Almonds	¼ cup	180	7	6	15
Olive Oil	1 tbsp	119	0	0	14
PB2 Peanut Butter	1 tbsp	23	3	3	1
Walnuts	¼ cup	195	4	4	18

Breakfast

Oatmeal with Fruit

- ½ cup oatmeal
- 1 scoop Beverly International Vanilla UMP Protein Powder
- ½ cup strawberries
- ¼ cup blueberries

Mix oatmeal with water and microwave until desired temperature. Stir in protein powder, add fruit and serve.

Per Serving:
Calories 289
Carbs 40g
Fat 5g
Protein 25g
Sugar 8g
Sodium 353mg

Chocolate Peanut Butter Oatmeal

- ½ cup dry oatmeal
- 1 scoop of Beverly International Chocolate UMP Protein Powder
- 2 tbsp PB2 Powdered Peanut Butter
- hot water

In a small bowl, mix oatmeal, protein powder and peanut butter. Add hot water to your desired consistency.

Makes 1 serving.

Per Serving:
Calories 315
Carbs 36g
Fat 9g
Protein 30g
Sugar 2g
Sodium 294mg

Blueberry Muffins

- 2 cups of egg whites
- 8 tbsp. of PB2 Powdered Peanut Butter
- 1 ½ cups oatmeal
- 2 scoops of Beverly International Vanilla UMP Protein Powder
- ½ cup unsweetened applesauce
- ¼ tsp baking soda (Bob's Red Mill Aluminum Free)
- 1/8 tsp baking powder
- 1 tsp vanilla extract
- 1 cup fresh blueberries

Mix all ingredients together except the blueberries. Spoon into muffin pan and then top each muffin with 3 – 4 blueberries. Bake at 350 for 15– 18 minutes.

Makes 12 muffins.

Per Serving:
Calories 106
Carbs   13 g
Fat 2g
Protein 11g
Sugar 3g
Sodium 155mg

Chocolate Peanut Butter Muffins

- 2 cups of egg whites or Muscle Egg Chocolate Egg Whites
- 8 tbsp PB2 Powdered Peanut Butter
- 1 ½ cups plain oatmeal
- 2 scoops of Beverly International Vanilla UMP Protein Powder
- ½ cup unsweetened applesauce
- ½ cup Walden Farms Chocolate Syrup
- ¼ tsp baking soda (Bob's Red Mill Aluminum Free)
- 1/8 tsp baking powder
- 1 tsp vanilla extract

Mix all ingredients together. Pour mixture into muffin pan. Bake at 350 for 15-18 minutes.

Makes 12 muffins

Per Serving:
Calories 98
Carbs   11 g
Fat 2g
Protein 11g
Sugar 2g
Sodium 161mg

Cookies n' Cream Pancakes

- 1 cup egg whites
- 1 cup oatmeal
- 1 tbsp Better than Peanut Butter*
- 1 scoop of Beverly International Cookies n' Cream UMP Protein Powder

Mix all ingredients and cook on griddle. Serve plain or use Walden Sugar Free Pancake Syrup and spray butter.

Makes 4 large pancakes.

Per Serving: (2 pancakes)
Calories 300g
Carbs 33g
Fat 5g
Protein 30g
Sugar 3g
Sodium 329mg

*You can substitute "Better than Peanut Butter" for 2 tbsp of PB2 Powdered Peanut Butter

Chocolate Pancakes

- 1 cup Muscle Egg Chocolate Egg Whites
- ½ cup oatmeal
- 1 scoop Beverly International Chocolate UMP Protein Powder
- 2 tbsp of Better than Peanut Butter

Mix all ingredients together. Cook on skillet sprayed with olive oil. Serve plain or with spray butter and sugar free syrup.

Makes 4 large pancakes.

Per Serving: (2 pancakes)
Calories 250
Carbs 25g
Fat 5g
Protein 27g
Sugar 2g
Sodium 374mg

Peanut Butter Pancakes

- 4 egg whites
- ½ cup oatmeal
- 2 tbsp of PB2 Powdered Peanut Butter or Better than Peanut Butter
- 1 tsp cinnamon
- 1 tsp Splenda

Mix all ingredients together. Spray griddle with fat free cooking spray and cook pancakes. Serve with Walden Farms Sugar Free Pancake Syrup & spray butter if desired.

Makes 4 small pancakes.

Per Serving: (4 pancakes)
Calories 217
Carbs 32g
Fat 5g
Protein 16g
Sugar 2g
Sodium 150mg

Strawberry Pancakes

- 1 cup egg whites
- ½ cup oatmeal
- 1 scoop Beverly International Vanilla UMP Protein Powder
- 2 packages of Stevia
- 1 tbsp cinnamon
- ½ cup fresh strawberries diced
- ½ cup fresh blueberries

Mix egg whites, oatmeal, protein powder, stevia and cinnamon. Add fruit and blend together. Cook on skillet sprayed with olive oil.
Serve with Walden Farms Sugar Free Pancake Syrup & spray butter if desired.

Makes 4 large pancakes.

Per Serving: (2 pancakes)
Calories 228
Carbs 26g
Fat 2g
Protein 29g
Sugar 8g
Sodium 223mg

Vanilla Apple Pancakes

- 1 cup Muscle Egg Vanilla Egg Whites
- ½ cup oatmeal
- ¼ cup homemade applesauce (see my recipe) or use organic unsweetened applesauce
- 1 tsp cinnamon

Mix all ingredients together. Cook on griddle sprayed with olive oil. Serve with a ¼ cup warm homemade applesauce on top.

Makes 8 small pancakes.

Per Serving: (4 small pancakes)
Calories 162
Carbs 21g
Fat 2g
Protein 16g
Sugar 4g
Sodium 201mg

Chocolate Mint Pancakes

- 1 cup Muscle Egg Mint Chocolate Egg Whites
- ¼ cup almond meal
- ¼ cup oatmeal
- 1 scoop Beverly International Chocolate UMP Protein Powder
- 1 tsp vanilla

Mix all ingredients and cook on griddle. Serve plain or use Walden Sugar Free Pancake Syrup and spray butter.

Makes 6 Pancakes.

Per Serving: (3 pancakes)
Calories 259
Carbs 15g
Fat 11g
Protein 28g
Sugar 2g
Sodium 300mg

Veggie Omelet

- 4 egg whites
- 1 whole egg
- 1/2 tbsp olive oil
- 1 cup of fresh veggies (spinach, onions, peppers, mushrooms & zucchini)

In small bowl, mix egg whites and whole egg together. In skillet, add olive oil and pour egg mixture. Add veggies, as eggs are cooking, fold into half to make omelet.

Makes 1 serving.

Per Serving:
Calories 223
Carbs 6g
Fat 12g
Protein 23g
Sugar 1g
Sodium 274mg

Chocolate French Toast

- 4 slices of whole wheat bread or P28 Bread
- 1 cup Muscle Egg's Chocolate Egg Whites
- 1 scoop of Beverly International Chocolate UMP Protein Powder
- 1 packet of Stevia
- 1 tsp cinnamon
- 1 tsp of vanilla extract

Mix egg whites, protein powder, Stevia, cinnamon & vanilla extract in bowl. Dip bread in bowl and cover both sides with mixture. Spray skillet with olive oil spray & cook until brown on each side. Serve with sugar free syrup.

Makes 4 servings.

Per Serving: (1 slice)
Calories 195
Carbs 15g
Fat 4g
Protein 26g
Sugar 4g
Sodium 360mg

French Toast with Maple Topping

- 6 slices of whole wheat bread or P28 Bread
- 1 cup egg whites
- ½ cup almond milk
- 2 packets of Stevia
- 1 tbsp cinnamon
- 1 tsp of vanilla extract

Mix egg whites, almond milk, Stevia, cinnamon & vanilla extract in bowl. Dip bread in bowl and cover both sides with mixture. Spray skillet with olive oil spray & cook until brown on each side.

Maple Topping:
- 4oz fat free cream cheese
- 1 scoop of Beverly International Vanilla UMP Protein Powder
- ¼ cup maple sugar free syrup
- ¼ cup almond milk
- walnuts (optional)

Mix cream cheese, protein powder, maple syrup & almond milk. Drizzle on top of French Toast. Sprinkle with walnuts if desired.

Makes 6 servings.

Per Serving: (1 slice with approx.. ¼ cup of maple topping)
Calories 202
Carbs 18g
Fat 5g
Protein 24g
Sugar 5g
Sodium 459mg

Breakfast Burrito

- 1 tsp extra virgin olive oil
- ½ cup ground turkey
- 1 tsp Mrs. Dash Southwestern Chipotle Seasoning
- ¼ cup green peppers – diced
- ¼ cup onions – diced
- ½ cup egg whites
- ¼ cup tomatoes - diced
- ¼ cup black beans –no salt
- 2 La Banderita whole wheat taco shells

Place turkey, chipotle seasoning, olive oil, green peppers and onions in skillet and brown until meat is cook. Add egg whites to mixture, stirring until egg whites are cooked. Add black beans & tomatoes. Serve on warm tortilla.

Makes 2 servings.

Per Serving: (1 shell with mixture)
Calories 286
Carbs 30g
Fat 10g
Protein 19g
Sugar 3g
Sodium 331mg

Sweet Potato Soufflé

- ¼ cup sweet potato diced
- 1 tsp cinnamon
- 1 tsp olive oil
- 1 cup egg whites (or vanilla egg whites)

In mini beanpot, add sweet potato, cinnamon & olive oil. Microwave for approx. 2 minutes until potatoes are tender. Pour in egg whites, cover with lid and microwave for another 2 ½ minutes.

Makes 1 serving.

Per Serving:
Calories 203
Carbs 14g
Fat 5g
Protein 26g
Sugar 1g
Sodium 429mg

Appetizers

Cinnamon Tortilla Crisps

- 4 Mama Lupe Low Carb Tortilla Shells
- fat free spray butter
- cinnamon
- stevia extract

Cut tortilla shells into quarters. Spray with fat free butter. Sprinkle with cinnamon & stevia extract. Bake on cookie sheet at 400 for 10 – 15 minutes or until crisp.

Note: Stevia extract looks like powdered sugar. (Trader Joes)

Serves 8

Per Serving: (2 crisps)
Calories 42
Carbs 5g
Fat 2g
Protein 4g
Sugar 0g
Sodium 156mg

Tortilla Chips

- 4 Mama Lupe Low Carb Tortilla Shells
- fat free spray butter

Cut tortilla shells into quarters. Spray with fat free spray butter. Bake on cookie sheet at 400 about 10 – 15 minutes or until crisp. Serve with Black Bean & Corn Salsa.

Serves 8.

Per Serving (2 Chips, doesn't include salsa):
Calories 38
Carbs 4g
Fat 2g
Protein 4g
Sugar 0g
Sodium 155mg

Guacamole

- 1 small avocado
- 4 tbsp fresh salsa
- 1 tbsp lemon juice
- 1 tbsp garlic powder
- 1 tbsp onion powder

Mix all ingredients together until avocado is blended. Chill & serve with my homemade tortilla chips.

Makes 8 servings.

Per Serving: (2 tbsp)
Calories 40
Carbs 2g
Fat 3g
Protein 1g
Sugar 1g
Sodium 12mg

Warm Chicken Dip

- 8oz chicken cooked & shredded
- 8oz fat free cream cheese
- 2 tbsp Mrs. Dash Fiesta lime seasoning
- ¼ cup fat free shredded cheese
- ¼ cup green onions
- 1 box of Blue Diamond Almond Nut-Thins

Mix cooked & shredded chicken with cream cheese, fiesta lime seasoning, shredded cheese and green onions. Warm dip. Serve with Nut-Thins.

Makes 16 servings.

Per Serving: (4 crackers with ½ tbsp. of dip on each cracker)
Calories 62
Carbs 7g
Fat 1g
Protein 6g
Sugar 1g
Sodium 159mg

Tuna Spread

- 1 package of low sodium tuna
- ¼ cup fat free cream cheese
- ¼ cup low fat cottage cheese
- 1 tbsp garlic powder
- 1 tsp black pepper
- ½ cup chopped green onion

Blend tuna, cream cheese, cottage cheese, garlic powder and pepper in blender. Add green onions and serve with veggies or crackers.

Makes 8 servings.

Per Serving: (2 tbsp)
Calories 27
Carbs 2g
Fat 0g
Protein 4g
Sugar 1g
Sodium 79mg

Tuna Salsa Dip

- 1 package low sodium tuna
- 4 tbsp fresh salsa
- 1 tsp extra virgin olive oil
- 1 tsp black pepper
- ½ avocado

Mix all ingredients together until avocado is blended. Chill & serve with veggies or crackers.

Makes 8 servings.

Per Serving: (2 tbsp)
Calories 40
Carbs 2g
Fat 3g
Protein 3g
Sugar 0g
Sodium 18mg

Dill Dip

- ½ cup fat free cream cheese
- ½ cup fat free sour cream
- 2 tsp dill seed
- ¼ tsp garlic powder

Mix all ingredients together. Chill & serve with crackers or veggies.

Makes 8 servings.

Per Serving: (2 tbsp)
Calories 29
Carbs 3g
Fat 0g
Protein 3g
Sugar 2g
Sodium 128mg

Taco Dip

- 8 oz fat free cream cheese
- 8 oz fat free sour cream
- 16 oz low sodium black bean & corn salsa or fresh salsa
- 1 tsp Mrs. Dash Chipotle Seasoning
- 1 tbsp chili powder
- 2 cups shredded lettuce
- 2 cups fresh diced tomatoes
- ½ cup green onions
- ½ cup fat free shredded cheddar cheese

Mix cream cheese, sour cream, salsa, chipotle seasoning and chili powder with mixer. Spread in 9 x 13 pan. Top with lettuce, tomatoes, onions and shredded cheese. Serve with homemade baked tortilla chips.

Serves 8

Per Serving: (does not include chips)
Calories 73
Carbs 9g
Fat 0g
Protein 8g
Sugar 7g
Sodium 333mg

Fruit Dip

- 2 cups plain 0% Greek yogurt
- 1 container fat free Cool Whip
- 4 Scoops Beverly International Vanilla UMP Protein Powder

Mix all ingredients. Chill & serve with fruit.

Per Serving: (4 tbsp)
Calories 88
Carbs 9g
Fat 1g
Protein 10g
Sugar 4g
Sodium 78mg

Chocolate Fruit Dip

- 1 cup Muscle Egg's Chocolate Egg Whites
- 2 scoops Beverly International Chocolate UMP Protein Powder
- 2 tbsp of PB2 Powder Peanut Butter

Mix all ingredients. Chill & serve with fruit.

Per Serving: (1/4 cup)
Calories 69
Carbs 3g
Fat 2g
Protein 12g
Sugar 0g
Sodium 149mg

Vanilla Peanut Butter Dip

- 1 cup plain egg whites
- 2 scoops Beverly International Vanilla UMP Protein Powder
- 2 tbsp PB2 Powdered Peanut Butter

Mix all ingredients together and serve with your favorite fruit like strawberries, bananas or apple slices.

Per Serving: (¼ cup serving)
Calories 68
Carbs 3g
Fat 1g
Protein 12g
Sugar 1g
Sodium 139 mg

Chicken Roll-Ups

- 8oz chicken cooked & shredded
- 8oz fat free cream cheese
- 2 tbsp Mrs. Dash Fiesta lime seasoning
- ¼ cup fat free shredded cheese
- ¼ cup green onions
- 6 La Banderita Fat Free Tortillas

Mix cooked & shredded chicken with cream cheese, fiesta lime seasoning, shredded cheese and green onions. Spread mixture over tortilla shells and roll. Cut the rolled tortilla shells into 12 pieces each. Chill & serve.

Makes 12 servings.

Per Serving: (6 pieces per serving)
Calories 95
Carbs 11g
Fat 0g
Protein 9g
Sugar 1g
Sodium 283mg

Veggie Pizza

- 1 whole grain thin pizza crust
- ¾ cup fat free cream cheese
- ¾ cup sour cream
- 3 tsp dill seed
- 1 tsp garlic powder
  2 cups fresh veggies of your choice (broccoli, cauliflower, cucumbers, onions, etc.

Bake pizza crust until crisp. Mix cream cheese, sour cream, dill seed and garlic powder together to make spread. Remove crust from oven & let cool. Spread mixture over bread and top with fresh veggies. Cut into 9 slices.

Makes 9 servings.

Per Serving:
Calories 170
Carbs 28g
Fat 2g
Protein 8g
Sugar 3g
Sodium 246mg

Fruit Pizza

- 1 P28 Flat Bread
- 5 sprays of "I Can't Believe It's Not Butter"
- 1 tbsp cinnamon
- 2 packets of Stevia
- 1 cup plain 0% Greek yogurt
- 1 cup fat free Cool Whip
- 1 scoop Beverly International Vanilla UMP Protein Powder
- 2 cups fresh fruit, cut (strawberries, blueberries, kiwi, pineapple, etc.)

Spray P28 flat bread with 5 sprays of butter and sprinkle cinnamon and stevia over flat bread. Bake until crisp. In a bowl mix yogurt, cool whip and vanilla protein powder. Remove bread from oven and let cool. Spread mixture on bread and top with fresh fruit. Cut into 9 squares.

Makes 9 servings.

Per Serving:
Calories 116
Carbs 18g
Fat 2g
Protein 6g
Sugar 8g
Sodium 73mg

Coconut Shrimp

- 12 oz. package jumbo shrimp cooked
- 1 tbsp coconut oil
- ½ cup unsweetened coconut
- 1 tbsp garlic powder

Place shrimp, coconut oil and unsweetened coconut in tortilla warmer. Sprinkle with garlic and microwave 10–13 minutes.

Serves 4

Per Serving:
Calories 141
Carbs 3g
Fat 8g
Protein 13g
Sugar 1g
Sodium 175mg

Italian Meatballs

- 2 lbs lean ground turkey or sirloin
- ½ cup chopped onion
- 1 tsp extra virgin olive oil
- 3 cloves garlic, minced
- ¼ cup fresh cilantro
- ½ cup fresh sweet basil
- ½ cup dry oatmeal
- 1/3 cup egg whites
- 6 tbsp parmesan cheese
- ¼ cup skim milk

Sauté onion and then mix with all other ingredients. Roll into 1-½ inch size balls. Bake on wire rack at 400 degrees for 12-15 minutes until done. Serve with spicy Italian sauce.

Makes about 50+ meatballs.

Per serving: (1 meatball)
Calories 30
Carbs 1g
Fat 1g
Protein 5g
Sugar 0g
Sodium 24mg

Spicy Italian Sauce

- 1 - 28 oz. can no salt crushed tomatoes (Del Fratelli)
- ½ cup yellow onion (chopped)
- 2 cloves of garlic
- 1 whole seeded jalapeno pepper (about 3 inch size)
- ¾ cup fresh sweet basil
- 2 packets stevia in the raw

Put all ingredients in food processor to chop and blend together. Simmer on stove until heated through and flavors blend together.

Per serving: (1/2 cup)
Calories 40
Carbs 8g
Fat 0g
Protein 2g
Sugar 6g
Sodium 25mg

Soups, Salads, Dressings & More

Chicken Enchilada Soup

- 2 large chicken breasts
- 1 container low sodium chicken broth (approx.4 cups of Trader Joes Chicken Broth)
- 1 can diced green chilies
- 1 can no salt Eden Organic Black Beans
- 1 can no salt diced tomatoes
- 2 cups frozen corn
- 2 tsp Mrs. Dash Southwest Chipotle Seasoning
- 4 tbsp chili powder
- 1 tbsp ground cumin
- 1 tbsp garlic powder
- 1 tsp turmeric
- 1 oz fresh cilantro
- 4 tbsp cream cheese
- black pepper to season
- fat free cheddar cheese
- fat free sour cream

Place chicken breasts in beanpot and microwave for 5 – 8 minutes. Take out and chop or shred chicken. Add chicken and remaining ingredients in beanpot and microwave 15 – 20 minutes. Serve with fat free cheddar cheese and fat free sour cream.

Serves 8

Per serving:
Calories 169
Carbs 23g
Fat 3g
Protein 12g
Sugar 4g
Sodium 173mg

Chicken Taco Chili

- 16oz. boneless chicken breasts
- 16oz. can low sodium black beans
- 16oz. can low sodium kidney beans
- 16oz. can no salt tomato sauce
- 16oz. can no salt diced tomatoes
- 2 tbsp chili powder
- 1 tbsp Mrs. Dash Chipotle Seasoning

Combine all ingredients in crockpot. Cook on high for 6 hours or low for 10 hours. Chicken should fall apart and shred with fork when done.

Recipe serves 8

Per serving: (approx.. 1 cup)
Calories 157
Carbs 22g
Fat 2g
Protein 15g
Sugar 5g
Sodium 125mg

White Chicken Chili

- 2 large chicken breast - chopped or shredded
- 1 container (4 cups) low sodium chicken broth
- 2 cans Eden Cannellini No Salt White Kidney Beans
- 1 can diced green chilies
- 2 green onions chopped
- 1 tbsp garlic powder
- 1 tsp ground cumin
- 1 tbsp dried oregano
- 1 oz. fresh cilantro - chopped
- 4oz fat free cream cheese
- 1 cup plain fat free Greek yogurt
- pepper to taste
- fat free mozzarella cheese (optional)
- fat free sour cream (optional)

Place chicken breast in beanpot. Microwave for 5-7 minutes until chicken is cooked. Chop or shred chicken. In a small bowl, mix together cream cheese and Greek yogurt together. Put all remaining ingredients in beanpot, add chicken and yogurt mixture. Microwave for 15 – 20 minutes until warm. Stir occasionally. Top with cheese and sour cream if desired.

Serves 8

Per Serving:
Calories 160
Carbs 20g
Fat 1g
Protein 18g
Sugar 3g
Sodium 273mg

Taco Soup

- 1 lb extra lean ground beef or ground turkey 96% - 99% fat free
- 1 tbsp extra virgin olive oil
- 2 tbsp chili powder
- 1 tbsp Mrs. Dash Southwest Chipotle
- 2 can no salt diced tomatoes
- 1 can no salt Eden Organic Black Beans
- 1 can no salt tomato sauce
- ½ package frozen corn
- fat free sour cream
- fat free cheddar cheese

Place ground beef or turkey, olive oil, chili powder, chipotle seasoning in beanpot. Microwave for 5-7 minutes until meat is browned. Add tomatoes, beans, tomato sauce and corn into beanpot. Microwave 15 minutes until heated. Serve with fat free sour cream and fat free cheddar cheese.

*Can also add in onions and peppers.

Serves 8

Per serving:
Calories 233
Carbs 28g
Fat 3g
Protein 26g
Sugar 5g
Sodium 67mg

Turkey Chili

- 1 lb fat free ground turkey breast (99% fat free)
- 1 tbsp olive oil
- 2 tbsp chili powder
- 1 tbsp Mrs. Dash Southwest Chipotle Seasoning
- ½ cup chopped onion
- 1 cup sliced red peppers
- ½ cup low sodium chicken broth
- 1 can no salt Eden Organic Kidney Beans
- 1 can no salt Eden Organic Black Beans
- 2 cans no salt diced tomatoes
- 1 can diced green chilies
- black pepper to taste
- fat free sour cream
- fat free shredded cheese

Place turkey, olive oil, chili powder and chipotle seasoning in beanpot. Microwave for 5-7 minutes until meat is browned. Add onions, sliced peppers and chicken broth into beanpot. Microwave for an additional 3 – 4 minutes. Add beans, tomatoes, green chilies and pepper. Microwave 10 – 15 minutes until warm. Serve with sour cream and cheese.

Serves 8

Per Serving:
Calories 218
Carbs 23g
Fat 3g
Protein 25g
Sugar 4g
Sodium 148mg

Beef Stew

- 1 lb lean stew meat
- 1 cup oatmeal (grind to flour consistency in blender)
- ¼ tsp black pepper
- 1 tsp Mrs. Dash original table blend
- 1 tsp garlic powder
- 2 tbsp extra virgin olive oil
- 4 cups low sodium beef broth (Pacific Organic broth is a great broth)
- 1 – 8 oz can no salt added tomato sauce
- 1 cup dry red wine
- 1 medium onion, chopped
- 2 stalks of celery, chopped
- ½ tsp thyme
- ½ tsp basil
- 3 carrots, sliced
- 1 small butternut squash
- ½ package of frozen peas (5 oz)
- ½ package of frozen green beans (5 oz)

Season oatmeal flour with pepper, Mrs. Dash and garlic powder. Heat olive oil in a dutch oven. Dredge stew meat in flour mixture and place in hot oil, brown for about 3-4 minutes. Add beef broth, tomato sauce, wine, onion, celery, thyme and basil to stew meat. Simmer for 30 minutes. Add carrots and continue to simmer until carrots become slightly tender. Add squash, peas and green beans until all vegetable are tender and liquids thicken to a gravy consistency.

Serves 8

Per Serving: (approx. 2 cups)
Calories 250
Carbs 27g
Fat 8g
Protein 16g
Sugar 6g
Sodium 248mg

Taco Salad

- 4 Joseph's Flax, Oat Bran and Whole Wheat Pita Bread
- 1lb extra lean ground turkey
- 1 tbsp chili powder
- ¼ cup water
- 15oz can no salt kidney beans – do not drain
- shredded lettuce
- 1 small chopped onion
- 1 small chopped green pepper
- 1 small chopped tomato
- 1 tbsp black bean and corn salsa
- 1 tbsp fat free sour cream (optional)
- 1 tbsp fat free Shredded Cheddar Cheese (optional)

Using medium size bowls, place the pita shell in bowl pressing to the shape of the bowl. Bake at 350 until crisp. 10 – 15 minutes.

In the meantime, place turkey with chili powder and water in the beanpot and microwave for 5 minutes or until turkey is browned. Add kidney beans (do not drain) and microwave an additional 5 minutes. Layer lettuce in shells, add turkey, onion, peppers, tomato and salsa. Add cheese and sour cream if desired.

Serves 4

Per Serving:
Calories 292
Carbs 29g
Fat 3g
Protein 40g
Sugar 6g
Sodium 550mg

Pasta Salad

- 14 oz box whole wheat pasta
- 1 cup broccoli
- ½ cup cherry tomato
- ½ cup green onions
- ½ cup red bell peppers
- ½ cup Italian dressing

Make pasta according to box directions. Cool and add remaining ingredients. Chill and serve.

Serves 8

Per Serving: (approx. ½ cup)
Calories 173
Carbs 40g
Fat 1g
Protein 6g
Sugar 3g
Sodium 133mg

Spinach Salad with Tuna

- 1 cup spinach
- 1 package low sodium tuna
- ½ cup grapes, halved
- ½ cup strawberries, halved
- 1 tbsp onions, diced
- 1 tbsp celery, diced
- 1 tbsp green peppers, diced

Layer spinach with all ingredients. Top with 2 tbsp of Balsamic Vinaigrette Dressing recipe.

Serves 1

Per Serving: (includes 2 tbsp of Balsamic Vinaigrette Dressing)
Calories 183
Carbs 20g
Fat 3g
Protein 19g
Sugar 14g
Sodium 89mg

Grilled Chicken Salad

- 4 oz grilled chicken breast, cut in strips
- 1 cup spinach or romaine lettuce
- 4 cherry tomatoes, halved
- ¼ cup cucumbers, chopped
- 1/8 cup green peppers, diced
- 1/8 cup red onions, diced
- 1/8 cup celery, diced
- 1/8 cup unsalted walnuts, chopped if desired

Grill chicken and cut into strips. Layer lettuce with chicken and remaining ingredients. Top with 2 tbsp of Raspberry Salad Dressing recipe.

Serves 1

Per Serving: (includes 2 tbsp of Raspberry Salad Dressing)
Calories 279
Carbs 18g
Fat 9g
Protein 33g
Sugar 11g
Sodium 84mg

Quinoa Salad

- 1 cup quinoa
- 2 cup water
- 2 tbsp extra virgin olive oil
- 4 tbsp lime juice
- 2 tsp ground cumin
- 2 tsp red pepper flakes
- 1 cup halved cherry tomatoes
- 1 can black beans – no salt, drained and rinsed
- 1 cup green onions, finely chopped
- ¼ cup cilantro
- black pepper to taste

Bring quinoa and water to a boil in a saucepan. Reduce heat, cover and simmer until quinoa is tender and water has been absorbed, approx. 10-15 minutes. Whisk olive oil, lime juice and red pepper flakes together in a bowl to make dressing. Combine quinoa, tomatoes, black beans and green onions together in a bowl. Pour dressing over quinoa mixture; toss to coat. Stir in cilantro; season with pepper. Serve immediately or chill in fridge.

Serves 6

Per Serving: (approx. 1 cup)
Calories 125
Carbs 15g
Fat 6g
Protein 4g
Sugar 1g
Sodium 11mg

Balsamic Vinaigrette Dressing

- 6 tbsp balsamic vinegar
- 2 tbsp extra virgin olive oil
- 2 cloves of garlic
- 1 packet of Stevia

Mix all ingredients and serve on salad.

Makes 6 servings.

Per Serving: (2 tbsp)
Calories 34
Carbs 4g
Fat 2g
Protein 0g
Sugar 3g
Sodium 1mg

Raspberry Salad Dressing

- ½ cup balsamic vinegar
- ½ cup plain 0% Greek yogurt
- 1 cup fresh raspberries
- ¼ cup water
- 2 packets of Stevia

Blend all ingredients in blender.

Makes 8 servings.

Per Serving: (2 tbsp)
Calories 36
Carbs 5g
Fat 0g
Protein 2g
Sugar 7g
Sodium 7mg

Sweet & Spicy Salad Dressing

- ¼ cup water
- 1 cup balsamic vinegar
- 1 tbsp honey Dijon mustard
- 2 tsp garlic powder
- ½ tsp pepper
- 2 packets of Stevia

Mix all ingredients together.

Makes 8 servings.

Per serving: (2 tbsp)
Calories 30
Carbs 8g
Fat 0g
Protein 0g
Sugar 6g
Sodium 42mg

Pasta/Pizza Sauce

- 1 can no salt diced tomato
- 1 can no salt tomato sauce
- 1 small onion
- 1 tbsp basil
- 1 tbsp onion powder
- 1 tbsp oregano
- 1/2 tbsp black pepper
- 1 tbsp parsley

Microwave:
Place all ingredients in beanpot. Microwave for 10 – 15 minutes.

Stove Top:
Place all ingredients in pan and simmer for 30 minutes.

Makes 6 servings.

Per Serving: (4 tbsp)
Calories 41
Carbs 9g
Fat 0g
Protein 1g
Sugar 4g
Sodium 28mg

BBQ Sauce

- 15oz can of no salt tomato sauce
- 4 tsp Worcestershire sauce
- 4 tsp organic brown sugar or Splenda Brown Sugar
- 1 tbsp red wine vinegar
- 1 tsp Mrs. Dash Southwest Chipotle
- 1 tsp onion powder
- 1 tsp garlic powder

In a small bowl, mix all ingredients to make the BBQ sauce.

Makes 8 servings.

Per Serving: (2 tbsp)
Calories 30
Carbs 7g
Fat 0g
Protein 0g
Sugar 5g
Sodium 50mg

Taco Seasoning

- 2 tsp chili powder
- 1 ½ tsp paprika
- 1 ¼ tsp ground cumin
- 1 tsp onion powder
- ¼ tsp garlic
- ¼ tsp cayenne pepper

Mix all spices together. To make taco meat, mix with 1lb of lean ground beef. Brown meat on skillet, adding 1 cup of water to the meat mixture.

Makes 1 serving.

Per Serving: (2 tbsp of taco seasoning only)
Calories 42
Carbs 9g
Fat 4g
Protein 1g
Sugar 1g
Sodium 56mg

Main Dish

Apple Pork Loin

- 1 lb lean pork tenderloin
- ¼ cup Braggs Organic Apple Cider Vinegar
- ½ cup unsweetened applesauce or homemade applesauce
- ½ cup organic low sodium chicken broth
- 1 tbsp cinnamon
- ½ tsp pumpkin pie spice
- ½ tsp apple pie spice
- 4 tsp Splenda Brown Sugar (optional)
- 1 medium apple - sliced

Place pork loin in beanpot, add vinegar, applesauce and chicken broth. Add the remaining ingredients and sliced apple on top. Bake at 350 for 1 ½ - 2 hours until pork is tender.

Serves 4

Per Serving:
Calories 193
Carbs 14g
Fat 4g
Protein 24g
Sugar 10g
Sodium 68mg

Braised Balsamic Pork Loin

- 6 boneless pork loin chops (4 oz)*
- 1 tsp garlic powder
- ground black pepper to taste
- 2 tbsp extra virgin olive oil
- 1 medium onion, thinly sliced
- ½ cup balsamic vinegar
- 1 can of no salt added diced tomatoes
- 1 tsp dried basil
- 1 tsp oregano
- 1 tsp dried rosemary
- ½ tsp dried thyme

Season pork loins with pepper and garlic powder. Heat olive oil in a medium skillet, and brown the onion and seasoned pork loins. Pour tomatoes and balsamic vinegar over pork loins, and season with basil, oregano, rosemary and thyme. Simmer until pork is cooked through.

*may substitute pork for chicken breasts.

Serves 6

Per Serving: (1 pork chop)
Calories 337
Carbs 10g
Fat 17g
Protein 35g
Sugar 7g
Sodium 80mg

Skillet Pork and Cabbage

- 6 – ½" sliced boneless pork loin chops (4oz)
- 2 tsp extra virgin olive oil
- 1 medium onion, thinly sliced
- 2 garlic cloves, minced
- 1 cup low sodium chicken broth, divided in ½ cups
- ½ tsp dried thyme
- ¼ tsp black pepper
- 4 cups coarsely shredded red or green cabbage
- 2 tbsp balsamic vinegar

In skillet, heat olive oil over medium heat for 30 seconds. Add pork chops in a single layer; flipping once until browned, approx. 2 minutes per side. Remove pork and set aside. (If necessary, cook pork chops in two batches).

Remove skillet from heat and coat with cooking spray. Add onion and garlic. Cook over medium heat until onion is translucent, stirring occasionally, about 5 minutes. Add ½ cup of broth to skillet; scrape up any browned bits of food with a wooden spoon. Stir in thyme and pepper. Return pork to skillet; sprinkle cabbage on top. Pour remaining ½ cup broth into skillet, cover and reduce heat to low. Simmer turning pork over and stirring cabbage halfway through cooking, about 45 minutes. Add vinegar during last 15 minutes of cooking time.

Serves 6

Per Serving: (1 pork chop & 2/3 cup of veggies)
Calories 299
Carbs 9g
Fat 13g
Protein 36g
Sugar 5g
Sodium 333mg

Shredded BBQ Pork

- 2lbs – 97% Fat Free Boneless Pork Loin
- 15oz can of no salt tomato sauce
- 4 tsp Worcestershire sauce
- 4 tsp organic brown sugar or Splenda Brown Sugar
- 1 tbsp red wine vinegar
- 1 tsp Mrs. Dash Southwest Chipotle
- 1 tsp onion powder
- 1 tsp garlic powder

Place pork in beanpot. In a small bowl, mix all remaining ingredients to make the BBQ sauce. Pour sauce over top of pork. Bake at 350 for 1½ hours until pork is tender. Or Microwave: cook in beanpot for 20-25 minutes until pork is tender and falls apart.

Serves 8

Per Serving:
Calories 152
Carbs 7g
Fat 2g
Protein 25g
Sugar 5g
Sodium 83mg

Chicken Salad Wrap

- 4 oz cooked & shredded chicken
- ¼ cup apples, diced
- ¼ cup grapes, halved
- ¼ cup celery, diced
- ½ cup plain 0% Greek yogurt
- 2 packets of Stevia
- ½ cup shredded lettuce
- 2 Mama Lupe low carb tortilla shells

Mix chicken, apples, grapes, celery, yogurt and Stevia together in bowl. Serve on tortillas with shredded lettuce.

Serves 2

Per Serving: (1 wrap)
Calories 171
Carbs 11g
Fat 4g
Protein 24g
Sugar 8g
Sodium 316mg

BBQ Chicken

- 2lbs of fat free chicken breast tenders
- 15oz can of no salt tomato sauce
- 4 tsp Worcestershire sauce
- 4 tsp organic brown sugar or Splenda Brown Sugar
- 1 tbsp red wine vinegar
- 1 tsp Mrs. Dash Southwest Chipotle
- 1 tsp onion powder
- 1 tsp garlic powder

Place chicken in beanpot. In a small bowl, mix all remaining ingredients to make the BBQ sauce. Pour sauce over top of chicken. Bake at 350 for 1½ hours until chicken is tender. Or Microwave: cook in beanpot for 20-25 minutes until chicken is tender.

Serves 8

Per Serving:
Calories 149
Carbs 7g
Fat 2g
Protein 27g
Sugar 5g
Sodium 116mg

Chicken Enchiladas

- 4 boneless, skinless chicken breasts
- ½ cup black bean and corn salsa
- 1 tbsp Mrs. Dash Southwestern Chipotle Seasoning
- ½ cup fat free sour cream
- ¼ cup fat free cheddar cheese
- 4 Buena Vida Low Carb Tortilla Shells

Place chicken, salsa and chipotle seasoning in beanpot. Microwave for 15 – 20 minutes until chicken is tender. Shred chicken and add sour cream and cheese. Microwave for an additional 3 minutes and serve on tortilla shells.

Serves 4

Per Serving: (approx. 1 cup of mixture) (does not include tortilla shell)
Calories 154
Carbs 5g
Fat 2g
Protein 29g
Sugar 3g
Sodium 245 mg

Chicken Fajitas

- 1lb boneless skinless chicken breast tenders
- 1 cup low sodium chicken broth
- 2 tsp Mrs. Dash Southwest Chipotle Seasoning
- 1 medium green pepper
- 1 medium red pepper
- 1 medium yellow pepper
- 1 medium onion
- 4 tbsp black bean and white corn salsa
- 4 tbsp fat free sour cream
- 4 tbsp fat free shredded cheddar cheese
- 4 Buena Vida Low Carb Tortilla Shells

Place chicken, broth, and chipotle seasoning in beanpot. Microwave for 10 minutes. Slice all vegetables and add to the beanpot microwave 10 more minutes or until vegetables are tender. Serve on low carb shell with 1 tbsp each of salsa, cheese and sour cream.

Serves 4

Per Serving: (includes cheese, tortilla shell, sour cream and salsa)
Calories 260
Carbs 17g
Fat 5g
Protein 36g
Sugar 3g
Sodium 487mg

Chicken Quesadilla

- 1 whole wheat tortilla
- 4 oz shredded chicken
- ¼ cup diced green onions
- ¼ cup fresh mushrooms
- ¼ cup spinach
- 2 tbsp fresh black bean and corn salsa
- 1 tbsp fat free cheese

Cook chicken and shred. Sautee onions, mushrooms and spinach until tender in skillet. Layer chicken, veggies, salsa and cheese in tortilla. Fold over and grilled in pan sprayed with olive oil turning 1 time. Grill until cheese is melted.

Serves 1

Per Serving:
Calories 248
Carbs 18g
Fat 5g
Protein 35g
Sugar 4g
Sodium 472mg

Lemon Pepper Chicken

- 6 boneless skinless chicken breast
- 1 container low sodium chicken broth
- 1 small onion sliced
- 1 large green bell pepper sliced
- 1 tbsp garlic powder
- 1 tbsp Mrs. Dash Lemon Pepper Seasoning

Place chicken breast in beanpot and add the remaining ingredients. Bake 350 for 1 – ½ hours until chicken is tender and falls apart.

Per Serving:
Calories 143
Carbs 5g
Fat 2g
Protein 27g
Sugar 7g
Sodium 100mg

Mexican Chicken

- 6 boneless skinless chicken breast
- 1 tsp Mrs. Dash Southwestern Chipotle
- 1 can black bean and corn salsa
- 1 can low sodium tomato sauce
- 1 small onion, sliced
- 1 large green bell pepper, sliced
- 1 large red pepper, sliced

Place chicken breast in beanpot and add the remaining ingredients. Bake 350 for 1 – 1½ hours until chicken is tender and falls apart.

Serves 6

Per Serving:
Calories 178
Carbs 13g
Fat 2g
Protein 27g
Sugar 7g
Sodium 356mg

Santa Fe Chicken

- 6 boneless skinless chicken breast
- 1 tsp Mrs. Dash Southwestern Chipotle Seasoning
- 15oz can low or no sodium diced tomatoes
- 1 can diced green chilies
- 15oz can Eden's Black Beans No Salt
- 1 package frozen corn
- 2 cups low sodium chicken broth
- ¼ c chopped fresh cilantro
- 1 tsp garlic powder
- 1 tsp onion powder

Place chicken breasts in beanpot and add the remaining ingredients. Bake 350 for 1½ hours until chicken is tender and falls apart.

Serves 6

Per Serving: (1 chicken breast)
Calories 275
Carbs 29g
Fat 3g
Protein 33g
Sugar 6g
Sodium 204mg

Southwest Chicken Marinade

- 4 fresh extra lean chicken breast
- 2 tbsp of Mrs. Dash Southwest Chipotle Marinade
- 1 cup fresh mushrooms
- 1/2 cup of diced red onions
- 2 tsp garlic
- 2 tsp black pepper

Place chicken in skillet first until browned on both sides. Add remaining ingredients and sauté until chicken and veggies are cooked thoroughly.

Serves 4

Per serving:
Calories 144
Carb 6g
Fat 2g
Protein 28g
Sugar 3g
Sodium 383mg

Pineapple Chicken

- 1 lb natural chicken breasts
- 8 oz water
- 4 tbsp Mrs. Dash Spicy Teriyaki Marinade
- 1 cup fresh pineapple
- ¼ cup chopped green onion
- 1 tbsp onion powder
- 1 tbsp garlic powder

Place all ingredients in beanpot. Bake in oven at 350 for 1 ½ hours or until chicken is tender.

Serves 4.

Per Serving (4oz chicken breast)
Calories 180
Carbs 13g
Fat 2g
Protein 27g
Sugar 8g
Sodium 53mg

BBQ Chicken Pizza (Individual)

- 1 Joseph's Flax Tortilla shell
- 2 tbsp Bone Suckin' BBQ sauce
- 4 oz shredded chicken
- 1/8 cup green peppers
- 1/8 cup onions
- 1/8 cup mushrooms
- 1 tbsp fat free shredded cheese

Pour BBQ sauce over tortilla shell. Add chicken, pepper, onion and mushroom. Top with cheese. Bake at 350 for 20 minutes on a cookie sheet.

Serves 1

Per Serving:
Calories 353
Carbs 26g
Fat 3g
Protein 32g
Sugar 10g
Sodium 772mg

Personal Pan Pizza

- 4 oz. cooked ground turkey breast (99% fat free)
- ¼ cup water
- 1 pita bread (Joseph's Flax, Oat Bran and Whole Wheat)
- 2 tbsp Southwest Black Bean and Corn Salsa
- ¼ cup chopped onions
- 1 tbsp fat free mozzarella cheese

Place ground turkey, Ms. Dash seasoning and ¼ cup water in beanpot. Microwave for 5-7 minutes until turkey is browned. Layer pita bread with salsa, turkey and onions or any other vegetables. Top with cheese. Bake at 350 for 10 – 15 minutes or until cheese is melted.

Per Serving: (1 pizza)
Calories 236
Carbs 16g
Fat 3g
Protein 38g
Sugar 3g
Sodium 623mg

Spaghetti

- 1lb ground turkey breast or extra lean ground beef – 97-99% fat free
- 1 tbsp olive oil
- 1 small onion
- 1 tbsp basil
- 1 tbsp onion powder
- 1 tbsp oregano
- 1/2 tbsp black pepper
- 1 can no salt diced tomato
- 1 can no salt tomato sauce
- 2 tbsp agave nectar
- 1 package whole wheat spaghetti noodles

Microwave:
In the beanpot, place turkey, olive oil, onion, basil, onion powder, oregano and pepper. Microwave for 5 – 8 minutes until meat is browned. Meanwhile, cook noodles on stove top and set aside. After the meat mixture is browned, add diced tomatoes, tomato sauce and agave nectar. Microwave an additional 5 minutes. Stir in cooked noodles microwave for 10 minutes.

Stove Top:
Place turkey, olive oil, onion, basil, onion powder, oregano and pepper in skillet and brown. Meanwhile, cook noodles on stove top and set aside. After the meat mixture is browned, add diced tomatoes, tomato sauce and agave nectar. Simmer for 25 minutes. Stir in cooked noodles or serve on top of cooked noodles.

Serves 6

Per Serving:
Calories 291
Carbs 29g
Fat 4g
Protein 35g
Sugar 7g
Sodium 302mg

Lasagna

- 1lb ground turkey breast - 99% fat free
- 1 tbsp olive oil
- 1 small onion
- 1 tbsp basil
- 1 tbsp onion powder
- 1 tbsp oregano
- 1 tsp black pepper
- 1 can no salt diced tomato
- 1 can no salt tomato sauce
- 6 whole wheat lasagna noodles
- 1 cup fat free cottage cheese
- ½ cup fat free mozzarella cheese
- pinch reduced fat parmesan cheese
- 1 tbsp parsley

Microwave:
In the beanpot, place turkey, olive oil, onion, basil, onion powder, oregano and pepper. Microwave for 5 – 8 minutes until meat is browned. Meanwhile, break lasagna noodles into 1/3 and cook on stove top and set aside. After the meat mixture is browned, add diced tomatoes and tomato sauce. Microwave an additional 5 minutes. Stir in cooked lasagna noodles and drop by spoon full the cottage cheese. Top with mozzarella cheese, parmesan cheese and parsley. Microwave for 10 minutes .

Oven:
Cook turkey, olive oil, onion, basil, onion powder, oregano and pepper in pan on stove until meat is browned. Meanwhile, cook lasagna noodles on stovetop. Set aside. Add diced tomatoes and tomato sauce to the meat mixture. In a 8x8 pan, pour 1/3 of meat sauce on bottom of pan, layer ½ the noodles, 1/3 of meat sauce, ½ cup of cottage cheese and repeat. Top with mozzarella cheese, parmesan cheese and parsley. Cover with foil & bake at 350 for 45 minutes.

Serves 6

Per Serving:
Calories 291
Carbs 29g
Fat 4g
Protein 35g
Sugar 7g
Sodium 302mg

Turkey Vegetable Lasagna

- 1 lb lean ground turkey (97-99% fat free)
- 1 small red onion, chopped
- 1 tbsp garlic powder
- 1 tsp dried oregano
- 1 tsp black pepper
- 1 can no salt tomato sauce
- 1 can no salt diced tomatoes
- 1 medium zucchini, chopped
- 1 medium yellow squash, chopped
- 1 container Ronzoni Healthy Harvest Whole Grain Lasagna Noodles (cooked and drained)
- 1 cup fat free cottage cheese
- 1 cup fat free mozzarella cheese
- reduced fat parmesan cheese *(optional)*

Place turkey, red onion, garlic powder, oregano and black pepper in beanpot. Microwave for 5-7 minutes until turkey is cooked thoroughly. Add tomato sauce, diced tomatoes, zucchini and squash. Microwave for an additional 5-10 minutes until veggies are cooked. Cook noodles as directed and drain.

Layer a 9x13 pan with 1/3 of the meat mixture, noodles and ½ cup of cottage cheese. Repeat. Layer top with 1 cup mozzarella cheese. Bake in oven 350 for 25 minutes, covered with foil. Remove and cool before cutting into 9 squares. Sprinkle parmesan cheese on top if desired.

Serves 9

Per Serving:
Calories 292
Carbs 41g
Fat 3g
Protein 30g
Sugar 6g
Sodium 358 mg

Zucchini Lasagna

- 1lb lean ground turkey (97-99% fat free)
- 1 small red onion, chopped
- 1 tbsp garlic powder
- 1 tsp dried oregano
- 1 tsp black pepper
- 1 can no salt tomato sauce
- 1 can no salt diced tomatoes
- 3 medium zucchini, sliced thin
- 1 cup fat free cottage cheese
- 1 cup fat free mozzarella cheese
- reduced fat parmesan cheese *(optional)*

Place turkey, red onion, garlic powder, oregano and black pepper in bean pot. Microwave for 5-7 minutes until turkey is cooked thoroughly. Add tomato sauce and diced tomatoes. Microwave for an additional 5-10 minutes until veggies are cooked.

In the meantime, slice the zucchini thin and lengthwise (to use as the "noodle") and grill zucchini on stove top. Blot with paper towel if needed.

Layer a 9x13 pan with 1/3 of the meat mixture, add layer of zucchini and ½ cup of cottage cheese. Repeat. Layer top with 1 cup mozzarella cheese. Cover with foil and bake in oven 350 for 25 minutes. Remove and cool before cutting into 9 squares. Sprinkle parmesan cheese on top if desired.

Serves 9

Per Serving:
Calories 168
Carbs 15g
Fat 1g
Protein 25g
Sugar 6g
Sodium 358 mg

Eggplant Parmesan with Chicken

- 6 slices of eggplant
- 6 - 4oz chicken breast (cooked)
- 6 slices of tomato
- 1 can no salt diced tomato
- 1 can no salt tomato sauce
- 1 small onion
- 1 tbsp basil
- 1 tbsp onion powder
- 1 tbsp oregano
- ½ tbsp black pepper
- 1 tbsp parsley
- 1 cup liquid egg whites
- 1 cup almond meal
- 1 tbsp garlic powder

To prepare sauce: (same as my pasta sauce recipe)
Microwave:
Place diced tomatoes, tomato sauce, onion, basil, onion powder, oregano and pepper and parsley in a beanpot. Microwave for 10 – 15 minutes.

Stove Top:
Place diced tomatoes, tomato sauce, onion, basil, onion powder, oregano and pepper and parsley in a pot. Simmer on stove top for 30 minutes.

To prepare eggplant:
Dip eggplant slices in egg whites then roll in almond meal. Sprinkle with garlic powder. Bake in 9x13 casserole for 20 minutes or until brown.

Layer:
Top each eggplant with a cooked chicken breast and a slice of tomato. Top with sauce. Add ¼ cup mozzarella cheese to each breast. Bake for 20 minutes at 350.

Serves 6

Per Serving:
Calories 334
Carbs 19g
Fat 11g
Protein 36g
Sugar 7g
Sodium 357mg

Fiesta Lime Avocado Turkey Burgers

- 1lb ground turkey 99% Fat Free
- Ms. Dash Fiesta Lime seasoning
- 1 avocado
- ½ cup black bean and corn salsa
- Sandwich Thins 100 calorie buns

Make 4 burgers and sprinkle with fiesta lime seasoning. Cook in skillet until done. Peel & dice avocado. In a small bowl, place avocado and salsa and mix together. Serve burgers with avocado/salsa mix on the sandwich thin buns.

Per Serving:
Calories 267
Carbs 26g
Fat 5g
Protein 33g
Sugar 5g
Sodium 318mg

Turkey Meatloaf Muffins

- 2lbs ground turkey
- 3 egg whites
- 1 cup oats
- ½ tsp ground cumin
- ½ tsp dried thyme
- 2 tsp dry yellow mustard
- 2 tsp black pepper
- 2 tsp chili powder
- 2 tbsp garlic powder (2 cloves, minced)
- 1 small onion, finely chopped
- 1 cup finely chopped celery

Preheat oven to 375. Spray muffin pan with olive oil spray. Mix all your ingredients together in a large mixing bowl. Roll mixture into 12 equal size balls and place in muffin pan. Bake for 40 minutes.

Serves 12

Per Serving: (1 muffin)
Calories 150
Carbs 7g
Fat 6g
Protein 16g
Sugar 1g
Sodium 84mg

Stuffed Green Peppers

- 4 large green peppers
- 1lb lean ground beef
- 1 cup cooked brown rice or quinoa
- 1 can no salt diced tomatoes
- 1 small onion
- 1 tbsp basil
- 1 tbsp parsley
- 1 tbsp garlic powder
- 1 tbsp oregano
- black pepper to taste
- fat free mozzarella cheese (optional)

Cut tops off green peppers and clean out inside. In a skillet, brown hamburger and drain. Add tomatoes, onion, basil, parsley, garlic powder, oregano and black pepper into hamburger. Simmer for 10 minutes. Add cooked rice into hamburger mixture. Fill each pepper and place peppers in 8x8 baking pan. Cover with foil and bake at 350 for 20 minutes. Then, top each pepper with ½ tbsp of fat free mozzarella cheese and bake uncovered for an additional 10 minutes.

Serves 4

Per Serving:
Calories 249
Carbs 24g
Fat 3g
Protein 30g
Sugar 6g
Sodium 161mg

Teriyaki Turkey Cutlets with Pineapple Salsa

- 1 lb turkey cutlets
- 1 cup low sodium chicken broth
- ½ cup Mrs. Dash Teriyaki Marinade
- 1 tsp ginger
- 1 tsp cumin
- 1 tsp turmeric

Place all ingredients in beanpot. Bake at 350 for 1 – 1 ½ hours in bean pot. Or cook in crockpot for 4-6 hours on low.
Serve with pineapple salsa over top. (recipe below).

Serves 4

Per Serving: (1-4oz turkey cutlet with ¾ cup pineapple salsa)
Calories 215
Carbs 21g
Fat 1g
Protein 26g
Sugar 15g
Sodium 291mg

Pineapple Salsa:
- 2 cups fresh pineapple, chopped
- ½ cup red peppers, diced
- 2 whole green onions, diced
- 2 tbsp green chiles
- 1 tbsp lime juice
- 1 tsp basil

Mix all ingredients together. Chill in fridge while cutlets are being cooked. Serve ¾ cup over each turkey cutlet.

Serves 4

Per Serving: (approx. ¾ cup)
Calories 49
Carbs 12g
Fat 0g
Protein 1g
Sugar 9g
Sodium 32mg

Taco Casserole

- 1lb extra lean ground beef
- 2 - 8oz cans no salt tomato sauce
- 1 small onion
- 1 tsp Mrs. Dash Southwest Chipotle
- 1 tsp garlic powder
- 1 tbsp chili powder
- 1 cup fat free sour cream
- ½ cup fat free cottage cheese
- ½ cup fat free cheddar cheese
- 2 Joseph's Flax, Oat Bran and Whole Wheat Pita Bread

Place ground beef & onion in beanpot. Microwave for 5-7 minutes until brown. Add tomato sauce, Mrs. Dash, garlic powder & chili powder.
In a small bowl, mix together sour cream and cottage cheese and set aside.
Cut pita bread into small chip size squares. Bake at 350 for 10 minutes until crisp.
In an 8x8 pan, layer meat mixture & baked chips. Top with sour cream mixture and cheese. Bake at 350 for 25–30 minutes.

Serves 6

Per Serving:
Calories 211
Carbs 19g
Fat 4g
Protein 24g
Sugar 8g
Sodium 425

Tortilla Pie

- 1 lb lean ground beef (96% +)
- 15oz can no salt diced petite tomatoes - drained
- 15oz can no salt black beans - drained
- 1 tbsp chili powder
- 1 tsp Mrs. Dash Southwest Chipotle Seasoning
- 4 low carb tortilla shells
- 1 cup diced green pepper
- 4 diced green onions
- 1 cup fresh mushrooms
- ¼ cup fat free mozzarella cheese

Place ground beef, chili powder and Mrs. Dash chipotle seasoning in beanpot. Microwave for 5 – 7 minutes until meat is browned. Drain tomato and black beans and stir into meat mixture.

In a pie plate, layer 1 tortilla shell then spoon ¼ of the meat mixture on top. Sprinkle 1/3 of the peppers, onions and mushrooms, then add tortilla shell and repeat until 3 layers are done. The last (top) layer, use the remaining meat mixture and sprinkle with mozzarella cheese. Bake at 350 for 30–45 minutes.

Serves 8

Per Serving: (1 slice)
Calories 162
Carbs 15g
Fat 4g
Protein 18g
Sugar 2g
Sodium 242mg

Sloppy Joes

- 1 lb 97%-99% lean ground beef
- ½ cup chopped onion
- ½ cup chopped celery
- 15oz can of no salt tomato sauce
- 4 tsp Worcestershire sauce
- 4 tsp organic brown sugar or Splenda Brown Sugar
- 1 tbsp red wine vinegar
- 1 tsp Mrs. Dash Southwest Chipotle
- 1 tsp onion powder
- 1 tsp garlic powder

Place ground beef, onion and celery in beanpot. Microwave for 5-7 minutes until beef is done. In a small bowl, mix all remaining ingredients to make the sauce. Pour sauce over top of beef. Microwave another 4-5 minutes until meat is warm.

Serves 8

Per Serving: (approximately ½ cup mixture) – Meat only
Calories 133
Carbs 6g
Fat 7g
Protein 11g
Sugar 5g
Sodium 207mg

Serve on 100 Calorie Sandwich Thins – 100% Whole Wheat

Per Serving: (1/2 cup mixture with sandwich thin bun)
Calories 145
Carbs 9g
Fat 7g
Protein 12g
Sugar 5g
Sodium 229mg

Beef Roast with Apples

- 24oz beef sirloin roast
- 1 tbsp garlic powder
- 1 small, chopped red onion
- 1 tbsp cinnamon
- 1 tsp apple pie spice
- 1 apple with skin, sliced
- 1-2 cups water

Add all ingredients to the beanpot. Bake in the oven at 350° for 3 ½ hours.

Makes 6 servings.

Per Serving: (4oz)
Calories 125
Carbs 5g
Fat 4g
Protein 17g
Sugar 3g
Sodium 37mg

Flank Steak with Veggies

- 1lb flank steak
- 2 cups black bean and corn salsa
- ½ cup diced green peppers
- ½ cup red peppers

Combine all ingredients in beanpot. Bake until tender at 350 for 1 ½ hours.

Serves 4

Per Serving:
Calories 300
Carbs 16g
Fat 9g
Protein 37g
Sugar 3g
Sodium 149mg

Beef Stir-fry

- 1 lb flank steak, cut into strips
- 1 tbsp extra virgin olive oil
- 1 tsp low sodium Worcestershire sauce
- 1 tbsp garlic powder
- 1 cup green pepper, cut into strips
- 1 cup red pepper, cut into strips
- ½ cup diced onions
- ½ cup sliced yellow squash
- ¼ cup low sodium vegetable broth or beef broth
- 1 tsp oregano

Brown steak strips in skillet with olive oil. Add remaining ingredients and cook until vegetables are tender.

Serves 4

Per Serving: (approx. 4 oz)
Calories 280
Carbs 8g
Fat 12g
Protein 33g
Sugar 4g
Sodium 89mg

Tuna Casserole

- 2 packages of low sodium tuna
- 1 cup cooked brown rice
- ¼ cup skim milk
- 1 cup egg whites
- ½ cup diced onions
- ½ cup mushrooms
- ½ cup fat free shredded cheese

Mix tuna, rice, milk, egg whites, onions and mushrooms together. Spread them in a 8x8 pan. Cover and bake at 350 for 15-20 minutes. Remove from oven, top with cheese and bake uncovered for 3-5 minutes until cheese melts.

Serves 4

Per Serving:
Calories 141
Carbs 13g
Fat 1g
Protein 20g
Sugar 2g
Sodium 273mg

Pineapple Tilapia and Asparagus

- 4oz tilapia filet
- 2 tbsp pineapple salsa
- 5-6 asparagus

Place tilapia in beanpot and layer with salsa and asparagus. Microwave for 5 minutes until filet is cooked. Season if necessary with black pepper or Ms. Dash

Per Serving:
Calories 152
Carbs 9g
Fat 3g
Protein 24g
Sugar 5g
Sodium 188mg

Shrimp Spaghetti

- 16oz shrimp, cooked
- 8oz whole wheat spaghetti
- 2 tbsp extra virgin olive oil
- 16oz Brussels sprouts, rinsed and sliced
- ½ tsp nutmeg
- ½ cup low fat parmesan cheese, grated
- 1 tsp crushed red pepper flakes
- black pepper to taste

Cook pasta according to package. Reserve one cup of drained water. Meanwhile, heat oil in a large pan. Sauté garlic until fragrant, but not brown. Add Brussels sprouts and nutmeg to pan. Cook until the sprouts become brighter in color, about 5 minutes. Add reserved cooking liquid from noodles, cheese and red pepper flakes and pepper to pan. Cook for 5 more minutes over medium heat. Add drained pasta and shrimp. Mix to combine and heat through.

Serves 4

Per Serving: (approx. 2 cups)
Calories 393
Carbs 45g
Fat 11g
Protein 34g
Sugar 3g
Sodium 338mg

Shrimp Enchiladas

- 1lb fresh shrimp (cooked and diced)*
- 1 cup fresh spinach chopped
- 2 cups black bean & corn salsa – low sodium
- 8oz fat free cream cheese
- 1 tbsp onion powder
- 1 tsp garlic powder
- ½ cup fat free cheese
- 6 fat free tortillas

In bowl, add shrimp, ½ cup salsa, spinach, onion powder, garlic powder and cream cheese. Mix until blended. Spoon ½ cup of mixture in each tortilla. Rollup and place with seam side down in 9x13 pan. Pour remaining salsa and shredded cheese over top. Cover and bake at 350 for 20 minutes.
*Can substitute shrimp for chicken

Serves 6

Per Serving:
Calories 255
Carbs 40g
Fat 2g
Protein 19g
Sugar 3g
Sodium 766mg

Shrimp and Brussels Sprouts

- 16oz bag of shrimp
- 4 cups Brussels sprouts
- 1 tbsp garlic powder
- 2 tbsp olive oil

Place in 9x13 pan and roast on 350 for 20 – 25 minutes until done. Serve over pasta with pasta sauce or roasted veggies.

Serves 6

Per Serving:
Calories 89
Carbs 4g
Fat 1g
Protein 16g
Sugar 1g
Sodium 408mg

Shrimp Tacos

- 16oz bag of shrimp
- 1 tbsp extra virgin olive oil
- 1oz fresh cilantro
- 1 tbsp minced garlic
- 1oz lime juice

Sauté shrimp in olive oil, add cilantro, garlic and lime juice. Serve on low carb pita shells or corn tortilla. Add lettuce, fresh salsa, avocado, fat free sour cream and fat free cheddar cheese

Serves 4

Per Serving: (Shrimp mixture only)
Calories 125
Carbs 2g
Fat 5g
Protein 18g
Sugar 0g
Sodium 129mg

Fish Tacos

- 4 tilapia filets cut into strips
- 1 tbsp extra virgin olive oil
- 1 tbsp Mrs. Dash Southwest Chipotle
- ½ tsp black pepper
- 1 cup lettuce
- 1 cup onions
- 2 tbsp fresh salsa
- 4 Buena Vida Low Carb tortilla shells

Pour olive oil in bottom of skillet, place tilapia strips in pan. Sprinkle with seasonings and grill until done. Serve in tortilla shell and top with lettuce, onions and salsa.

Serves 4

Per Serving:
Calories 235
Carbs 12g
Fat 8g
Protein 25g
Sugar 2g
Sodium 298mg

Teriyaki Salmon Filets with Pineapple

- 4 oz salmon filet
- 1 tbsp Mrs. Dash Teriyaki marinade
- 1 tsp ginger
- 1 slice fresh pineapple

Marinate salmon in ginger and Mrs. Dash marinade for at least 15 minutes. Grill both the salmon and pineapple slice until tender. Serve pineapple on top.

Serves 1

Per Serving:
Calories 162
Carbs 9g
Fat 4g
Protein 19g
Sugar 4g
Sodium 66mg

Sweet Salmon Filets

- 4 oz salmon filet
- ½ tbsp agave nectar

Brush agave nectar on each side of filet. Grill in skillet until cooked.

Serves 1

Per Serving:
Calories 142
Carbs 8g
Fat 3g
Protein 19g
Sugar 8g
Sodium 65mg

Side Dish

Mashed Cauliflower

- 1 medium cauliflower head
- 1/3 cup fat free milk
- 1/3 cup fat free cream cheese
- pepper to taste
- garlic powder to taste

Steam or boil cauliflower until tender. Add remaining ingredients and mash.

Serves 8

Per Serving:
Calories 31
Carbs 4g
Fat 0g
Protein 3g
Sugar 3g
Sodium 72mg

Mashed Sweet Potatoes

- 4 sweet potatoes
- ½ cup unsweetened almond breeze
- 2 tbsp of cinnamon

Bake sweet potatoes at 350 for 45-60 minutes in oven. Remove from oven and scoop out potato from shells. In a small bowl, mash potato, almond breeze and cinnamon.

Makes 4 servings.

Per Serving: (1 cup)
Calories 61
Carbs 15g
Fat 0g
Protein 1g
Sugar 2g
Sodium 54mg

Sweet Potatoes

- 6 medium sweet potatoes
- 2 tbsp cinnamon
- 1 tbsp extra virgin olive oil

Peel and dice potatoes. Place in beanpot and top with cinnamon and olive oil. Stir until potatoes are well coated. Microwave for 15 minutes until potatoes are tender.

Serves 6

Per Serving: (1 medium potato)
Calories 112
Carbs 22g
Fat 2g
Protein 2g
Sugar 4g
Sodium 1mg

Spicy Sweet Potato Wedges

- 4 medium sweet potatoes
- 1 tbsp extra virgin olive oil
- 1 tbsp chili powder
- 2 tsp Mrs. Dash Chipotle Seasoning

Cut potatoes into wedges approx. 4 wedges per potato. Throw potato wedges and remaining ingredients into large zip lock bag. Shake in bag to cover wedges with seasonings. Place on cookie sheet and bake at 350 for 40-45 minutes or until tender.

Serves 4

Per Serving: (4 wedges)
Calories 193
Carbs 20g
Fat 2g
Protein 2g
Sugar 1g
Sodium 234mg

Sweet Potato Fries

- 4 medium sweet potatoes
- 1 tbsp extra virgin olive oil
- 2 tbsp cinnamon

Cut potatoes lengthwise into fries, approx. 8 fries per potato. Throw potato fries and remaining ingredients into large zip lock bag. Shake in bag to cover fries with seasonings. Place on cookie sheet and bake at 350 for 40-45 minutes or until tender.

Serves 4

Per Serving: (4oz serving)
Calories 150
Carbs 29g
Fat 4g
Protein 2g
Sugar 6g
Sodium 73mg

Roasted Brussels Sprouts & Sweet Potatoes

- 1 cup Brussels sprouts
- 1 cup sweet potatoes
- 2 tbsp extra virgin olive oil
- 2 tsp garlic powder

Coat veggies with olive oil and spread on cookie sheet. Sprinkle with garlic powder. Bake at 350 for 25-30 minutes until veggies are tender.

Serves 4

Per Serving: (approx. 1 cup)
Calories 122
Carbs 14g
Fat 7g
Protein 2g
Sugar 3g
Sodium 39mg

Quinoa with Black Beans

- ¾ cup quinoa, cooked
- 1 ¼ cup water
- 2 tsp extra virgin olive oil
- ½ cup chopped red onion
- ¾ cup frozen corn
- 1 can black beans – no salt, drained and rinsed
- 1 cup cherry tomatoes, quartered
- 1 tsp ground cumin
- 1 tsp chili powder
- 4 tbsp lime juice
- ¾ cup of reduced fat feta cheese
- ¼ cup fresh cilantro leaves
- black pepper to taste

Bring water to a boil in a saucepan. Stir in quinoa. Reduce the heat to low, cover and simmer until quinoa is cooked through, but still firm to the bite and the water is evaporated, 15 to 18 minutes. Remove from the heat, leave covered for 10 minutes.

Heat oil in skillet on medium heat and sauté the onion. Add the corn and cook approx. 2 minutes, then add bean and cook until heated through. Transfer to a large bowl. Add the quinoa, tomatoes, cumin, chili powder and lime juice, stir gently to combine. Stir in feta and cilantro and season to taste with black pepper.

Serves 6

Per Serving: (approx. 1 cup)
Calories 161
Carbs 22g
Fat 5g
Protein 9g
Sugar 2g
Sodium 248mg

Quinoa with Sun-Dried Tomatoes

- 2 cups quinoa
- 6 cups low sodium chicken broth
- 1 cup sun-dried tomatoes
- 1 tbsp garlic powder
- 1 medium green onion, chopped

In saucepan, bring broth, tomatoes, garlic powder and green onions to a boil. Add quinoa and cook until tender. Reduce heat, cover and cook until broth is absorbed.

Makes 4 servings.

Per Serving: (approx.1/2 cup)
Calories 154
Carbs 24g
Fat 2g
Protein 8g
Sugar 1g
Sodium 127mg

Cous Cous & Veggies

- 1 ½ cups chicken broth – low sodium
- 1 cup whole wheat cous cous
- 2 tsp onion powder
- ½ tsp garlic powder
- ½ tsp ground cumin
- ¾ cup frozen peas
- 1 can no salt diced tomatoes
- 2 tsp cilantro

Cook cous cous in chicken broth following directions on box. Add remaining ingredients and simmer for 5-10 minutes.

Serves 4

Per Serving: (approx. 1/2 cup)
Calories 217
Carbs 42g
Fat 1g
Protein 9g
Sugar 6g
Sodium 68mg

Rice Pilaf with Veggies

- 2 cups brown rice
- 2 cups low sodium chicken broth
- 1 cup diced carrots
- 1 cup frozen peas
- ½ cup chopped green onions

Beanpot:
Place everything in beanpot and microwave until veggies are tender for approx. 10 minutes.

Stove Top:
Place in pot on stove and bring to boil and simmer until veggies are tender.

Makes 8 Servings

Per Serving: (1/2 cup)
Calories 97
Carbs 21g
Fat 1g
Protein 3g
Sugar 1g
Sodium 32mg

Roasted Zucchini & Yellow Squash

- 2 medium zucchini, sliced
- 2 medium yellow squash, sliced
- 1 tbsp olive oil
- 1 tbsp garlic powder
- black pepper to taste

Slice zucchini and squash. Place in large zip lock bag with oil and spices to coat. Lay out on cookie sheet and bake at 350 for 20-25 minutes until veggies are tender.

Serves 4

Per Serving: (1 cup)
Calories 68
Carbs 7g
Fat 4g
Protein 3g
Sugar 5g
Sodium 20mg

Eggplant Casserole

- 1 cup eggplant cubed
- 1 cup zucchini (with skin) cubed
- 1 cup yellow squash (with skin) cubed
- 1 cup diced onion
- 1 cup diced green pepper
- 1 tbsp. black pepper
- 1tbsp garlic powder
- 1 tbsp. parmesan cheese

Prepare eggplant, zucchini, squash, onion and green pepper as directed above. Layer in a 9x13 casserole dish sprayed with olive oil. Add seasonings and mix. Bake at 350 for 30 minutes or until veggies are tender.

Makes 4 servings.

Per Serving: 2 cups
Calories 52
Carbs 11g
Fat 1g
Protein 3g
Sugar 5g
Sodium 32mg

Asparagus, Brussels Sprouts & Broccoli

- 2 cups fresh asparagus – cut into 3" pieces
- 2 cups Brussels sprouts – halved
- 2 cups broccoli florets
- 4 tbsp extra virgin olive oil
- 1 tbsp garlic powder
- black pepper to taste

Heat olive oil in skillet, add veggies and seasonings. Grill until veggies are tender and serve.

Serves 6

Per Serving: (1 cup serving)
Calories 117
Carbs 5g
Fat 10g
Protein 3g
Sugar 2g
Sodium 66mg

Grilled Asparagus

- 4 cups fresh asparagus, trimmed
- 1 tbsp chopped garlic
- 2 tsp fresh ground pepper
- 4 tsp extra virgin olive oil

Set up grill for direct cooking over medium heat and oil the grates. Place the trimmed asparagus on a baking sheet. Add the chopped garlic and pepper. Drizzle with olive oil, toss to coat. Place on grill directly or in a grill basket. Grill until just tender and lightly charred. About 5 minutes.

Serves 4

Per serving: (1 cup)
Calories 76
Carbs 4g
Fat 5g
Protein 2g
Sugar 2g
Sodium 1mg

Garlic Sautéed Spinach

- 8 cups fresh spinach
- 1 tbsp extra virgin olive oil
- 2 tsp chopped garlic cloves
- black pepper to taste
- 1 oz lemon juice

In skillet, sauté garlic cloves with olive oil. Add spinach and season with black pepper to taste. Once spinach is cooked, top off with lemon juice.

Serves 4

Per Serving: (1 – 1 ½ cups)
Calories 54
Carbs 2g
Fat 4g
Protein 2g
Sugar 0g
Sodium 65mg

Spaghetti Squash and Veggies

- 1 medium spaghetti squash
- 1 cup low sodium chicken broth
- 1 cup carrots chopped
- 1 cup green onion chopped
- 1 cup green pepper chopped
- 1 tsp black pepper
- 1 tbsp garlic powder

Prepare spaghetti squash and scoop out. Add to skillet and sauté with chicken broth and all remaining ingredients. Simmer until veggies are tender.

Serves 6

Per serving: (1 cup)
Calories 58
Carbs 13g
Fat 1 g
Protein 2g
Sugar 3g
Sodium 48mg

Sauté Green Beans, Squash & Onions

- 2 cups fresh green beans
- 1 cup water
- 1/4 cup red onions
- 1/2 medium size yellow squash
- 1 tsp garlic
- 1 tsp pepper

Place green beans & water in the beanpot. Cook for 10 minutes in microwave. Remove and place all ingredients in skillet and grilled until all veggies are cooked through.

Serves 4

Per Serving: (3/4 cup)
Calories 22
Carb 5g
Fat 0g
Protein 2g
Sugar 3g
Sodium 7mg

Italian Green Beans

- 1 lb. fresh green beans
- 1 lb. 97% lean ground turkey
- 1 small onion diced
- 3 cloves of garlic diced
- ½ tbsp. black pepper
- 1 can no salt diced tomatoes with basil, garlic & oregano
- 1 can no salt tomato sauce
- 1 tbsp. Worcestershire sauce
- ¼ cup reduced fat grated parmesan cheese

Snap ends off green beans and boil for approximately 10 minutes. Drain green beans and place in bottom of 8" x 8" baking dish. Brown turkey, onion, garlic, and pepper in a skillet. Add diced tomatoes, tomato sauce, and Worcestershire sauce and let simmer for 5 minutes. Layer meat mixture over top of green beans and sprinkle with parmesan cheese. Bake at 350° for 30 minutes.

Serves 9

Per Serving:
Calories 115
Carbs 11g
Fat 2g
Protein 13g
Sugar 4g
Sodium 107mg

BBQ Green Beans

- 1 package of frozen green beans
- 1 tsp. garlic powder
- 1tbsp olive oil
- ½ cup onion chopped
- 1 small can of Hunt's Tomato Paste (no salt added)
- 1 tbsp Worcestershire sauce
- 1 tbsp red wine vinegar
- 2 tsp organic brown sugar

In saucepan, add green beans, garlic powder, olive oil and onion. Heat on low, stirring occasionally. Add the remaining ingredients and let simmer until green beans are tender, about 20 minutes.

Serves 4

Per serving: (1 cup)
Calories 119
Carbs 18g
Fat 4g
Protein 3g
Sugar 11g
Sodium 68mg

Green Beans & Mushrooms

- 3 cups fresh or frozen green beans
- 1 cup fresh mushrooms, diced
- 1 cup green onions, chopped
- 1 tbsp extra virgin olive oil
- garlic powder to taste
- black pepper to taste

Steam green beans in microwave until tender. In skillet, sauté mushrooms, onions, oil and seasonings. Add green beans to skillet. Cook until veggies are tender and warm.

Serves 4

Per Serving: (1 cup serving)
Calories 83
Carbs 12g
Fat 4g
Protein 4g
Sugar 3g
Sodium 4mg

Kale Chips

- 1 package kale
- 2 tbsp olive oil
- 1 tbsp garlic powder
- black pepper to taste

Layer kale out on a cookie sheet. Drizzle olive oil and seasonings over kale. Bake at 350 for 10-15 minutes until crispy and slightly browned.

Serves 4

Per Serving: (1 cup)
Calories 100
Carbs 8g
Fat 7g
Protein 3g
Sugar 1g
Sodium 30mg

Applesauce

- 6 large apples
- 2 tbsp cinnamon
- 1 tbsp apple pie spice
- 1 tsp nutmeg
- 1 cup of water
- Stevia optional

Peel & dice apples. Place all ingredients in beanpot. Bake at 200 overnight.

Makes 18 servings

Per Serving: (1/4 cup)
Calories 20
Carbs 6g
Fat 0
Protein 0
Sugar 4g
Sodium 1mg

Desserts

Apple Oatmeal Cake

- 1 cup plain oatmeal
- 2 cups water
- 1 cup almond meal
- ½ cup egg whites
- 2 medium apples diced
- ½ tsp baking powder
- 1 tsp baking soda
- 1 tbsp cinnamon
- 1 tsp apple pie spice
- 4 tbsp Torani Sugar Free Caramel Syrup
- 2 tbsp Walden Farms Calorie Free Caramel Dip
- 5 scoops Beverly International Vanilla UMP Protein Powder

Mix all ingredients together. Bake at 350 in 9x13 pan for 30 minutes.

Serves 15

Per Serving:
Calories 123
Carbs 9g
Fat 5g
Protein 10g
Sugar 3g
Sodium 94mg

Brownies

- 1 box sugar-free Pillsbury Brownie Mix
- 3 scoops Beverly International Chocolate UMP Protein Powder
- 3 tbsp PB2 Powdered Peanut Butter
- 1 can 100% pure pumpkin
- ½ cup water

Mix all ingredients together. Bake in 9x13 pan at 350 for 25 minutes. Let cool. Cut into 15 squares.

Serves 15

Per Serving: (1 brownie)
Calories 110
Carbs 22g
Fat 3g
Protein 6g
Sugar 1g
Sodium 118g

Chocolate Almond Bars

- 1 cup almond butter unsalted
- ½ cup Almond Breeze Almond Milk Unsweetened
- 1 cup egg whites
- 2 tsp vanilla extract
- 1 cup almond meal
- 2 tbsp ground flaxseed
- ¼ tsp baking powder (Clabber Girl Double acting Gluten Free)
- ¼ tsp baking soda aluminum free
- 2 scoops Beverly International Vanilla UMP Protein Powder
- 2 packets stevia
- ¼ cup sugar free maple syrup
- 4 tbsp Organic Cacao Chocolate Chips

Mix almond butter, almond milk, egg whites and vanilla extract together. Add the remaining ingredients and stir. Pour mixture into a 9x13 pan sprayed with olive oil cooking spray.
Bake at 350 for 15 minutes.

Icing:

- 1 scoop of Beverly International Vanilla UMP Protein Powder
- ¼ cup sugar free maple syrup
- 2 tbsp fat free cream cheese

Mix all ingredients together until smooth. While bars are still warm, spread icing over top and serve.

Makes 15 bars

Per Serving:
Calories 153
Carbs 7g
Fat 10g
Protein 10g
Sugar 2g
Sodium 120mg

Chocolate Peanut Butter Cookies

- 3 scoops Beverly International Chocolate UMP Protein Powder
- 1 cup oats
- ½ cup almond meal
- ¼ cup slivered almond
- 4 packages stevia in the raw
- ¼ tsp baking soda aluminum free
- 1/4 tsp baking powder
- 2 cups egg whites
- 1 cup 100% pure pumpkin
- ½ cup Better than Peanut Butter

Mix all dry ingredients then add remaining ingredients. Drop by spoonful and bake on cookie sheet for 12 – 15 minutes at 350.

Makes 24 cookies

Per Serving:
Calories 72
Carbs 6g
Fat 3g
Protein 6g
Sugar 1g
Sodium 77mg

Chocolate Fudge

4 scoops Beverly International Chocolate UMP Protein Powder
4 tbsp Better than Peanut Butter
1 cup water

Mix peanut butter and protein powder and slowly add water. Batter needs to be thick.. Press in 8x8 pan and freeze for 30 minutes. Cut into 9 squares and then store in refrigerator.

Per Serving: (1 bar)
Calories 76
Carbs 5g
Fat 2g
Protein 10g
Sugar 0g
Sodium 110mg

Chocolate Peanut Butter Brownies

- 2 cups Muscle Egg's Chocolate Caramel Egg Whites
- 2 cups oatmeal
- 4 scoops Beverly International Chocolate UMP Protein Powder
- ½ cup organic unsweetened applesauce
- ½ cup Better than Peanut Butter
- 2 tbsp unsweetened cocoa
- ½ cup plain 0% Greek yogurt
- 1 tsp baking soda (low sodium)
- For sweetener use stevia drops (chocolate) optional

Mix together and spread in 9x13 pan. Bake at 350 for 25 minutes.

Makes 15 brownies.

Per Serving:
Calories 127
Carbs 14g
Fat 2g
Protein 12g
Sugar 2g
Sodium 207mg

Chocolate Coconut Bars

- 2 cups oatmeal
- 6 scoops Beverly International Chocolate UMP Protein Powder
- 1 cup Better Than Peanut Butter
- 1 cup water
- 1 cup unsweetened coconut
- ½ cup Walden Farms Sugar Free Pancake Syrup

Mix together all ingredients. Press in 9x13 pan. Freeze for 30 minutes. Cut into 18 squares and store in individual plastic zip lock baggie. Keep in freezer or refrigerator.

Makes 18 bars

Per Serving: (1 bar)
Calories 111
Carbs 11g
Fats 4g
Protein 9g
Sugar 1g
Sodium 98mg

Chocolate Peanut Butter Balls

- 2 scoops of Beverly International Chocolate UMP Protein Powder
- 2 tbsp sugar free, fat free instant pudding (Cheese Cake)
- ¼ cup oatmeal
- 4 tbsp Better N Peanut Butter
- ½ cup water

In bowl, place protein powder, instant pudding, oatmeal and peanut butter. Slowly add the water and mix until the mixture turns into dough. Roll into quarter size balls and lay on cookie sheet. Chill for at least and hour or until hard.

Makes 8 -10 Balls

Per Serving: (4 balls)
Calories 91
Carbs 9
Fat 2g
Protein 7g
Sugar 1g
Sodium 149mg

Caramel Apple Crisp

- 2 medium apples
- 4 tbsp Torani Sugar Free Caramel Syrup
- 2 tbsp Walden Farms Caramel Dip
- 1/2 cup Just Almond Meal (Trader Joe's)
- ½ cup Fiber One Original Bran Cereal
- 2 tbsp "I Can't believe its not Butter Light"

Slice up apples and place in 8 x 8 pan. Stir in caramel syrup and caramel dip. Microwave for 5 minutes, until apples are tender. In the meantime, grind up Fiber One bran cereal in blender. Mix together the blended bran cereal with almond meal and sprinkle on top of apples. Drizzle with melted "I Can't believe its not Butter". Bake at 350 for 10-15 minutes.

Serves 9

Per Serving:
Calories 69
Carbs 7g
Fat 5g
Protein 2g
Sugar 3g
Sodium 28mg

Caramel Apple Tacos

- 4 medium apples
- 4 tbsp Torani Sugar Free Caramel Syrup
- 1 cup water
- 8 tbsp cinnamon
- 2 tsp apple pie spice
- 4 scoops Beverly International Vanilla UMP Protein Powder
- Stevia
- 8 Low Carb Mama Lupe's Tortilla Shells

Slice apples and place in beanpot. Add sugar free syrup, water, cinnamon and apple pie spice. Microwave for 10 - 15 minutes (until apples are tender). Stir in protein powder. Fill each shell with the apple mixture, fold over and press to seal. Sprinkle with stevia and cinnamon. Bake at 350 for 15 - 18 minutes in 9 x 13 pan.

Serves 8

Per Serving (approx. 1 cup)
Calories 130
Carbs 17g
Fat 3g
Protein 13g
Sugar 1g
Sodium 216mg

Caramel Oatmeal Apple Bake

- 1 cup oatmeal
- 2 cups water
- ½ cup egg whites
- 2 medium apples diced
- ½ tsp baking powder
- 1 tbsp cinnamon
- 1 tsp apple pie spice
- 4 tbsp Torani Sugar Free Caramel Syrup
- 2 tbsp Walden Farms Calorie Free Caramel Dip
- 4 scoops Beverly International Vanilla UMP Protein Powder

Mix all ingredients together. Bake at 350 in beanpot for 45 minutes.

Serves 8

Per Serving:
Calories 125
Carbs 14g
Fat 2g
Protein 13g
Sugar 5g
Sodium 146mg

Chocolate Protein Bar and Apple Salad

- 3 5:1 Chocolate Covered Pretzel Protein Bars
- 3 medium apples
- 1 cup plain 0% Greek yogurt
- 1 container of fat free Cool Whip
- 6 Scoops Beverly International Vanilla UMP Protein Powder

Chop apples and protein bars. In a small bowl, mix yogurt, Cool Whip and protein powder with mixer. Stir in apples and bars. Chill and serve.

Serves 16.

Per Serving:
Calories 145
Carbs 14g
Fat 3g
Protein 15g
Sugar 6g
Sodium 116mg

Mint Chocolate Bars

- 2 cups oatmeal
- 3 scoops Beverly International Chocolate UMP Protein Powder
- 1 cup Better Than Peanut Butter
- 1 1/2 cup Muscle Egg's Mint Chocolate Brownie Egg Whites

Mix together all ingredients and press in 9x13 pan. Freeze for 30 minutes. Cut into 18 squares and store in zip lock baggies (1 square per baggie). Store in freezer or refrigerator.

Makes 18 bars.

Per Serving: (1 bar)
Calories 121
Carbs 14g
Fats 2g
Protein 9g
Sugar 1g
Sodium 131mg

Coconut Cupcakes

- 1 ½ cups Bob Red Mill Coconut Flour
- 2 scoops Beverly International Vanilla UMP Protein Powder
- 1 tsp aluminum free baking soda
- 1 cup organic brown sugar
- 1 cup plain 0% Greek yogurt
- 1 cup Muscle Egg's Vanilla Egg Whites
- 1 cup unsweetened almond breeze (vanilla or chocolate flavor)
- 1 tsp vanilla extract
- 4 packages of stevia (optional)

Mix all ingredients together. Spoon into muffin pan. Bake at 350 for 18-20 minutes.

Makes 18 cupcakes or 48 mini muffins.

Per Serving: (no icing)
Calories 111
Carbs 18g
Fat 2g
Protein 6g
Sugar 12g
Sodium 136mg

Icing:

- 1 Scoop Beverly International Vanilla UMP Protein Powder
- ¼ cup sugar free maple syrup
- 2 tbsp fat free cream cheese
- 1 tsp coconut extract
- unsweetened coconut (for garnish)

Mix together protein powder, syrup, cream cheese and extract until smooth. Top each cupcake with icing and garnish with coconut.

No Bake Cookies

- 1 cup oatmeal
- 1 cup hot water
- 3 scoops of Beverly International Chocolate UMP Protein Powder
- 2 tbsp Better than Peanut Butter

Mix oatmeal with hot water. Then add protein powder and peanut butter. Drop by spoonful on cookies sheet. Refrigerate overnight.

Makes 18 cookies.

Per Serving: (1 cookie)
Calories 42
Carbs 4g
Fats 1g
Protein 4g
Sugar 0g
Sodium 39mg

Oatmeal Apple Bake

- 1 cup oatmeal
- 2 cups water
- ½ cup egg whites
- 2 medium apples, diced
- ½ tsp baking powder
- 1 tbsp cinnamon
- 1 tsp apple pie spice
- 4 tbsp Torani Sugar Free Caramel Syrup
- 2 tbsp Walden Farms Calorie Free Caramel Dip

Mix all ingredients together. Bake at 350 in beanpot for 45 minutes.

Serves 8

Per Serving:
Calories 65
Carbs 14g
Fat 1g
Protein 3g
Sugar 4g
Sodium 61mg

Oatmeal Peanut Butter Bars

- 2 cups oatmeal
- 6 scoops Beverly International Vanilla UMP Protein Powder
- 1 cup Muscle Egg's Vanilla Egg Whites
- ½ cup water
- 4 tbsp Better Than Peanut Butter

Mix all ingredients together. Spread in 9x13 baker sprayed with olive oil. Freeze for 30 minutes. Cut into 15 squares. Store in refrigerator.

Makes 15 bars.

Per Serving: (1 bar)
Calories 109
Carbs 11g
Fat 2g
Protein 12g
Sugar 1g
Sodium 107mg

Peanut Butter Brownies

- 1 box Vita Top Muffin Mix
- 1 can 100% pure pumpkin
- 1½ cup egg whites
- 1 cup plain 0% Greek yogurt
- 4 tbsp Better than Peanut Butter

Mix muffin mix, pumpkin, egg whites and Greek yogurt together. Spread in 9x13 pan. Bake at 350 for 15-18 minutes. Top with peanut butter and cut into 15 squares.

Makes 15 brownies.

Per Serving: (1 brownie)
Calories 110
Carbs 21 g
Fat 1 g
Protein 8g
Sugar 8g
Sodium 142 mg

Pumpkin Cake

- 2 cups of oatmeal
- 6 scoops of Beverly International Vanilla UMP Protein Powder
- 15oz can 100% pure pumpkin
- 4 tsp cinnamon
- ¼ tsp nutmeg
- 1 tsp pumpkin pie spice
- 1 tsp aluminum free baking soda
- 2 ½ cups liquid egg whites
- 2 cups fat free plain 0% Greek yogurt
- 5 packets of Stevia (optional)
- ½ cup unsalted chopped walnuts

Blend oatmeal in blender until flour consistency. Then, add protein powder, pure pumpkin, cinnamon, nutmeg, pumpkin pie spice, baking soda, egg whites, yogurt and Stevia. Spread in 9x13 pan. Top with chopped walnuts. Bake at 350 for 30-35 minutes.

Serves 18

Per Serving:
Calories 138
Carbs 11g
Fat 4g
Protein 15 g
Sugar 4g
Sodium 196 mg

Pumpkin Oatmeal Bars

- 2 cups of oatmeal
- 6 scoops Beverly International Vanilla UMP Protein Powder
- 15oz can of pumpkin
- 1/8 tsp baking powder
- 1/8 tsp baking soda
- 1 tsp cinnamon
- 1 cup egg whites
- 1 cup water
- ½ cup almond meal
- ¼ cup flax seed meal
- 1 tsp vanilla
- ½ cup of unsalted chopped walnuts

Mix all ingredients together except the walnuts. Spread in 9x13 pan. Top with chopped walnuts. Bake at 350 for about 20 minutes. Cool and cut into 15 bars.

Makes 15 bars

Per Serving: (1 bar)
Calories 163
Carbs 13g
Fats 7g
Protein 13g
Sugar 2g
Sodium 120mg

Pumpkin Pie Cheesecake

- 8oz - 100% pure pumpkin
- 1 cup fat free plain 0% Greek yogurt
- 4 scoops Beverly International Vanilla UMP Protein Powder
- ¼ cup liquid egg whites
- 4oz of fat free cool whip
- 1 tbsp cinnamon

Mix all ingredients together with mixer and spread on crust and chill at least 1 hour.

Serves 8

Homemade Crust:
- ½ cup Fiber One Cereal
- ½ cup unsalted slivered almonds
- 2 tbsp extra virgin olive oil

Blend cereal and almond in blender. Add olive oil and press in bottom of pie pan. Bake at 350 for 15 minutes.

Per Serving: (1 slice) with homemade crust
Calories 154
Carbs 8g
Fat 9g
Protein 14g
Sugar 2g
Sodium 117mg

Graham Cracker Crust:
I like the Keebler Reduced Fat Graham Cracker Crust

Per Serving: (1 slice) with graham cracker crust
Calories 210
Carbs 25g
Fat 5g
Protein 14g
Sugar 10g
Sodium 212mg

Pumpkin Mousse

- 15oz can of pumpkin
- 1 cup Almond Breeze unsweetened
- 4 scoops Beverly International Vanilla UMP Protein Powder*
- 2 cups fat free plain 0% Greek yogurt
- 1 tbsp cinnamon
- 1 tbsp pumpkin pie spice
- 4 packets of Stevia
- 1 tsp vanilla extract

Mix all together in blender. Chill for at least 1 hour before serving.
*Can substitute vanilla protein for chocolate protein powder

Serves 12

Per Serving: (1/2 cup)
Calories 79
Carbs 6g
Fat 2g
Protein 11g
Sugar 3g
Sodium 98mg

Pumpkin Cupcakes with Icing

- 1 package of Pillsbury Sugar Free Yellow Cake Mix
- 15oz can of 100% pumpkin
- ½ cup Muscle Egg's Pumpkin Spice Egg Whites or regular egg whites
- ½ cup water
- 1 tsp cinnamon (add more if you used regular egg whites)

Mix all ingredients. Pour into cupcake pan. Bake at 350 for 15-20 mins.

Icing

- 2 scoops Beverly International Vanilla UMP Protein Powder
- ½ cup Muscle Egg's Pumpkin Spice Egg Whites or regular egg whites

Stir in egg whites slowly until it becomes thick like icing.

Serves 24

Per Serving: 1 cupcake
Calories 83
Carbs 17g
Fat 2g
Protein 4g
Sugar 1g
Sodium 172mg

Strawberry Fruit Tarts

- 6 Joseph's Flax, Oat Bran and Whole Wheat Pita Bread – Small
- cinnamon
- stevia extract powder
- ½ cup liquid egg whites
- 1 cup fat free plain 0% Greek yogurt
- 1 tsp strawberry imitation extract
- 4 tbsp fat free cream cheese (plain or strawberry)
- 2 scoops Beverly International Vanilla UMP Protein Powder
- 1 tsp Stevia
- 4 large strawberries
- ¼ cup Bare Naked Fruit and Nut Granola

Spray muffin pan with cooking spray. Brush each pita with liquid egg whites and sprinkle with cinnamon and stevia extract powder. Press each one in the muffin pan. Bake 350 for 20 minutes or until crispy. Let cool.

Mix yogurt, extract, strawberry pie ball, cream cheese, protein powder and stevia until smooth and creamy. When shells are cooled, spoon mixture in each shell. Top each one with sliced strawberries and garnish with granola. Refrigerate 30 minutes before serving.

Serves 6

Per Serving:
Calories 166
Carbs 19g
Fat 4g
Protein 18g
Sugar 6g
Sodium 400mg

Vanilla Peanut Butter Mini Cheesecakes

- ½ cup Fiber One Original Bran Cereal
- ½ cup slivered unsalted almonds
- 2 tbsp extra virgin olive oil
- 1½ cup plain 0% Greek yogurt
- 1 cup plain liquid egg whites
- 4 tbsp of PB2 Powdered Peanut Butter
- 1 container fat free cool whip topping
- 6 scoops Beverly International Vanilla UMP Protein Powder

Crust:
Grind up bran cereal and almonds in blender. Mix together with olive oil. Press crust mixture in mini cupcake pan. Bake at 350 for 15 - 20 minutes.

Filling:
Using a mixer, mix together yogurt, egg whites, powdered peanut butter, cool whip and protein powder.

Fill each crust with 1 scoop of filling mixture. Refrigerate for at least 1 hour before serving.

Makes 18 servings.

Per Serving: (1 mini cheesecake)
Calories 120
Carbs 10g
Fats 4g
Protein 11g
Sugar 3g
Sodium 111mg

White Chocolate Peanut Butter Bars with Vanilla Icing

- 1 cup oatmeal
- 3 scoops Beverly International Vanilla UMP Protein Powder
- 1 cup of PB2 Powdered Peanut Butter
- 1 cup liquid egg whites
- 1 cup of water
- 1/8 tsp baking powder
- ¼ tsp baking soda aluminum free
- 2 tbsp white chocolate Sugar Free Torani Syrup
- ¼ cup Splenda (optional)

Stir all ingredients in bowl. Spread in 9 x13 baker. Bake at 350 for 15 minutes.

Icing:

- 6 scoops of Beverly International Vanilla UMP Protein Powder
- ½ cup egg whites
- 2 tbsp white chocolate Sugar Free Torani Syrup
- 2 tbsp fat free cream cheese
- 1 tsp cinnamon
- water as needed

Blend all ingredients and add water as needed to desired thicknesses. When bars are cooled, ice with vanilla icing. Cut into squares and store in refrigerator in single serving plastic bags. They may be frozen too.

Makes 18 Bars.

Per Serving: (1 bar)
Calories 131
Carbs 10g
Fat 3g
Protein 17g
Sugar 2g
Sodium 228 mg

Blueberry Cookies

- ¾ cup liquid egg whites
- ½ cup oatmeal
- 2 scoops of Beverly International Vanilla UMP Protein Powder
- 2 tsp pure vanilla
- 1 tsp cinnamon
- ½ tsp baking powder
- 1 ½ tbsp. ground flaxseed
- 1 medium ripe banana
- 1 cup fresh blueberries

Mix all together. Bake on parchment paper in oven at 375 for approximately 9-10 minutes. Don't over bake.

Makes 20 cookies.

Per Serving: (1 cookie)
Calories 37
Carbs 4g
Fat 1g
Protein 3g
Sugar 2g
Sodium 45mg

Rocky Road Protein Bars

- 2 cups oats
- 4 scoops Beverly International Rocky Road UMP Protein Powder
- 1 tbsp unsweetened cocoa powder
- 6 tbsp Walden Farms Marshmallow Cream
- 6 tbsp Trader Joe's Almond Butter
- ¾ cup water

Combine oats, protein powder, and cocoa powder then add remaining ingredients; mixture will appear thick. Pour into 8x8 pan. Freeze for 30 minutes then thaw slightly and cut into 9 squares.

Make 9 bars.

Per serving:
Calories 184
Carbs 14g
Fat 9g
Protein 14g
Sugar 1g
Sodium 106mg

Rocky Road Brownies

- 1 cup oats
- 5 scoops Beverly International Rocky Road UMP Protein Powder
- 1 tsp baking soda
- 2 tbsp cocoa powder
- 2 tbsp Truvia
- ½ cup Walden Farms Marshmallow Cream
- 2 tbsp Trader Joe's Almond Butter
- ½ cup water
- 1 tsp vanilla extract
- ½ cup egg whites
- 1 cup unsweetened, organic apple sauce

Mix all dry ingredients then add in wet ingredients. Pour in lightly greased 9x13 pan. Bake at 350° for 18-20 minutes. Let cool and cut into 18 squares.

Makes 18 brownies.

Per Serving:
Calories 80
Carbs 6g
Fat 2g
Protein 9g
Sugar 2g
Sodium 176mg

Chewy Protein Bites

- 1 cup oats
- 2 scoops Beverly International Vanilla UMP Protein Powder
- ½ cup ground flaxseed
- ½ cup Better n Peanut Butter Low Sodium
- 1 cup unsweetened coconut flakes
- 1 ½ tsp vanilla extract

Mix all ingredients and roll into 1" balls. Keep refrigerated.

Makes 35 servings.

Per Serving: (1 ball)
Calories 39
Carbs 3g
Fat 2g
Protein 2g
Sugar 0g
Sodium 20mg

Conversion Chart

Unit:	Equals:	Also equals:
1 tsp.	1/6 fl. oz.	1/3 tbsp.
1 tbsp.	½ fl. oz.	3 tsp.
1/8 cup	1 fl. oz.	2 tbsp.
¼ cup	2 fl. oz.	4 tbsp.
1/3 cup	2¾ fl. oz.	¼ cup plus 4 tsp.
½ cup	4 fl. oz.	8 tbsp.
1 cup	8 fl. oz.	½ pint
1 pint	16 fl. oz.	2 cups
1 quart	32 fl. oz.	2 pints
1 liter	34 fl. oz.	1 quart plus ¼ cup
1 gallon	128 fl. oz.	4 quarts

Our Favorite Products

Cooking Products, Healthy Foods & Workout Programs

Check out the below links for some of our recommendations that you will find throughout our cookbook. Plus, some of our workout programs to help you achieve your fitness goals!

The **Beanpot** is a cooking dish that we love! The taste of a slow cooker, but much quicker cooking time! www.celebratinghome.com

NETRITION - http://www.netrition.com/cgi/goto.cgi?aid=3507
Beverly International Protein Powder
Bell Plantation PB2 Powdered Peanut Butter
Better N' Peanut Butter – Low Sodium
Better N' Peanut Butter – Chocolate
P28 Bread
P28 Flat Bread
P28 Bagels
Mama Lupe's Tortilla Low-Carb Shell
Walden Farm's Jelly
Walden Farm's Dressings (in moderation)
Walden Farm's Chocolate Syrup
Joseph's Sugar Free Maple Syrup
DaVinci Sugar Free Syrup

MUSCLE EGG
http://www.shareasale.com/r.cfm?B=326741&U=503340&M=35134&urllink=
Flavored Egg Whites – Vanilla, Chocolate, Chocolate Caramel, Strawberry and Mint Brownie – great to drink or cook with!

Get Fit in 4: The 28-Day Challenge - Our 28 day workout program
available on www.amazon.com or www.getfitmoms.com

Get Fit & Fabulous at Any Age – Nutritional Guide – Our complete
nutritional guide with all the tools to help you reach your goals!
www.amazon.com or www.getfitmoms.com

Get Fit & Fabulous at Any Age – Workout Program - Our workout
program for all fitness levels that requires very little equipment!
www.amazon.com or www.getfitmoms.com

For more great tips, products, workouts and recipes, check us out on Facebook at Get Fit Moms or www.getfitmoms.com